SEXUAL HEALTH AWARENESS

What Is

Gonorrhea?

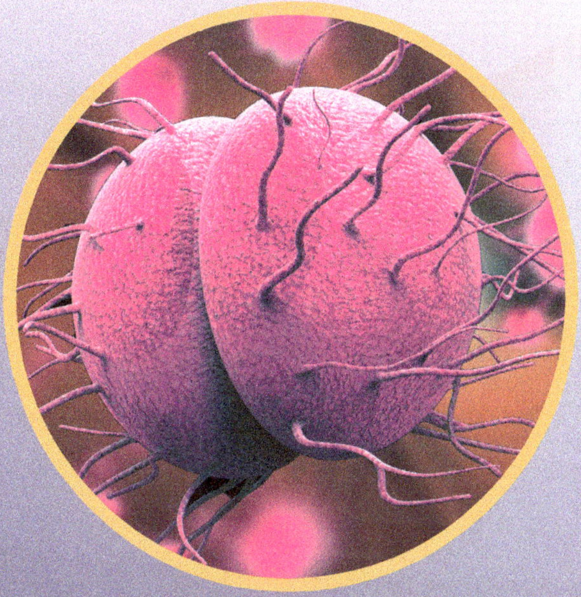

Sadie Silva

ROSEN PUBLISHING

NEW YORK

Published in 2022 by The Rosen Publishing Group, Inc.
29 East 21st Street, New York, NY 10010

First Edition

Portions of this work were originally authored by Tamra Orr and published as *Gonorrhea.* All new material in this edition was authored by Sadie Silva.

Library of Congress Cataloging-in-Publication Data

Names: Silva, Sadie, author.
Title: What is gonorrhea? / Sadie Silva.
Description: New York : Rosen Publishing, [2022] | Series: Sexual health awareness | Includes index. | Description based on print version record and CIP data provided by publisher.
Identifiers: LCCN 2021031851 (print) | LCCN 2021031852 (ebook) | ISBN 9781499472257 | ISBN 9781499472240 (paperback) | 9781499472264 (ebook)
Subjects: LCSH: Gonorrhea.
Classification: LCC RC202 (ebook) | LCC RC202 .S55 2022 (print) | DDC 616.95/15--dc23
Manufactured in the United States of America

CPSIA Compliance Information: Batch #CWRYA22. For further information contact Rosen Publishing, New York, New York at 1-800-237-9932.

CONTENTS

INTRODUCTION

Sexually transmitted infections (STIs) are common health issues, and their symptoms can range from annoying to very serious if left untreated. The Centers for Disease Control and Prevention (CDC) report that 1 in 5 people are dealing with an STI in the United States. And young people aren't immune to getting them. In fact, half of all STI cases are reported in people aged 15 to 24 years old. STIs can affect your sexual health, so it's important to learn as much as you can about what they are and how to prevent them.

Common STIs include HPV, chlamydia, HIV, and gonorrhea. Gonorrhea accounts for about 1.6 million new infections in the United States each year. In 2018, gonorrhea caused $271 million in direct medical costs. People who contract this infection deal with genital pain that can also cause missed days of school and work.

Gonorrhea is nothing new. In fact, it's one of the oldest known types of STI in history. For much of history, the bacterium that causes gonorrhea was unknown, and because of that, it was untreatable. But today, gonorrhea is completely curable. The bad news is that curing it is becoming more challenging because of people's increasing use of antibiotics, which makes bacteria more resistant to the effects of antibiotics. The bacterium that causes gonorrhea, *Neisseria gonorrhoeae*, is complex and adaptable. Once treated by a certain type of antibiotic, the gonorrhea bacteria will not respond to it again. Because of antibiotics and sexual health education, the rate of gonorrhea dropped dramatically between 1975 and 1997, hitting a record low in 2009. However, since then, it has slowly begun to rise again. By 2017–2018, rates of gonorrhea had gone up 82.6 percent since that 2009 low.

Fortunately, as with many STIs, gonorrhea is preventable. Sexual activity is the greatest risk factor for contracting gonorrhea. Choosing your sexual partner wisely and being open to communication and testing can help decrease your chances of contracting an STI like gonorrhea. Learning about other precautions and preventative behaviors can also help protect you from gonorrhea and show you how to take responsibility for your sexual health.

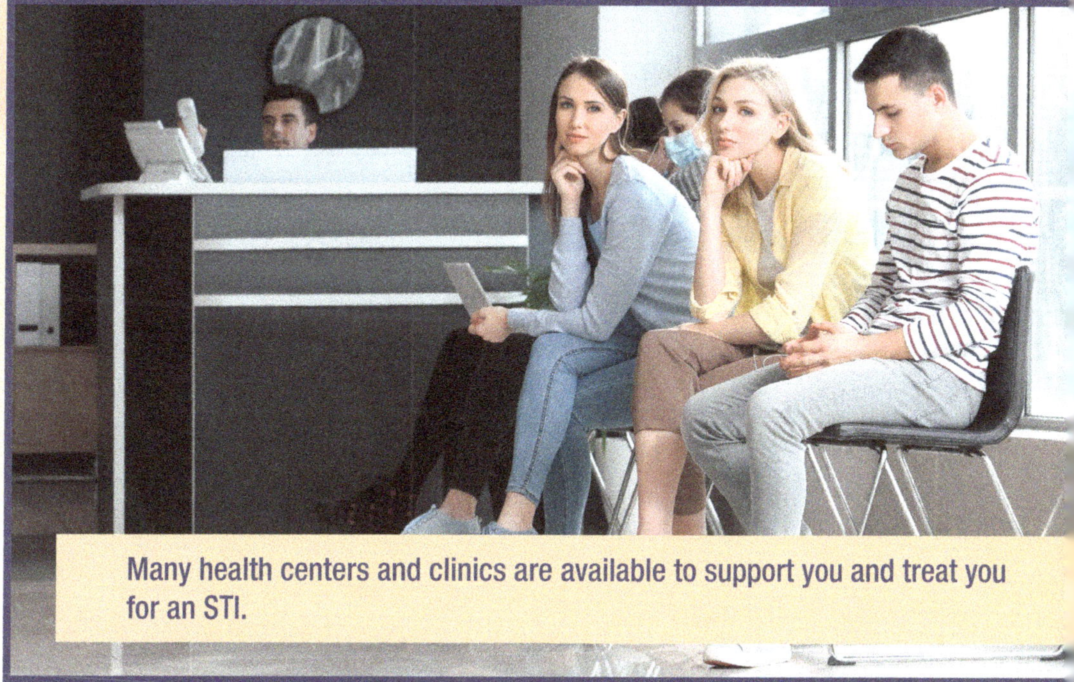

Many health centers and clinics are available to support you and treat you for an STI.

If you do test positive for gonorrhea, you can still get the treatment and support you need. Some people feel ashamed or embarrassed when they contract an STI, because there's often a stigma around sexual activity. However, no matter how someone gets gonorrhea, they deserve to get the care and medicine they need to get better. Doctors and other medical professionals are able to treat this STI fairly easily, especially if it's caught early.

Gonorrhea can impact people of any biological sex and gender identity. However, it's important to know how STIs like gonorrhea can affect you based on your assigned sex at birth (a label based on your hormones, chromosomes, and genitals at birth) or the body parts that you have. That's because those genetic, hormonal, and anatomical factors will play a role in how gonorrhea affects you and what your symptoms, and risks are.

The most powerful tool against gonorrhea is knowledge. The more you know, the more power you have to prevent, treat, and deal with an STI. Taking control of your sexual health is one of the challenges—and necessities—of becoming sexually active.

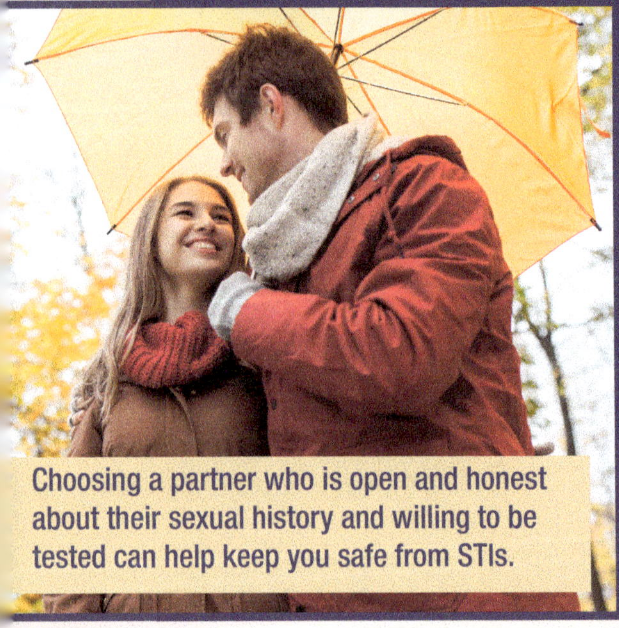

Choosing a partner who is open and honest about their sexual history and willing to be tested can help keep you safe from STIs.

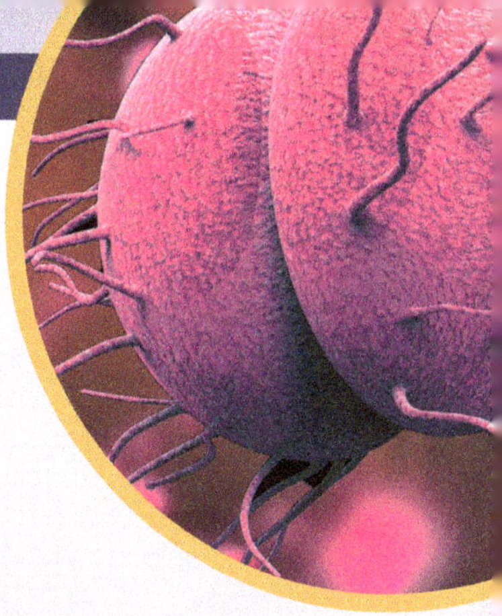

CHAPTER 1

GONORRHEA, PAST AND PRESENT

People have lived with gonorrhea for thousands of years. It's one of the oldest STIs known among humans. Although its origins aren't completely known, mentions of this sexually transmitted infection have been found in ancient writings. Medical professionals and researchers can use knowledge from the past to figure out how to treat, and how not to treat, this painful infection.

THE HISTORY OF GONORRHEA

When was the first case of gonorrhea recorded? Some researchers say it was mentioned in Chinese and Middle Eastern cultures more than 4,000 years ago. Records from that time period mention a disease that sounds a great deal like gonorrhea. In 2600 BCE, Chinese emperor Huang Ti described a condition that resembled gonorrhea. Even the Old Testament in the Bible refers to an issue of "seed" (semen) that could be gonorrhea. The book of Leviticus gives precautions one could take so as not to contract it. The disease finally got a name when the Greek physician Galen (131–200 CE) put together the Greek words for "semen" (*gonos*) and "to flow" (*rhoia*) to create the name "gonorrhea."

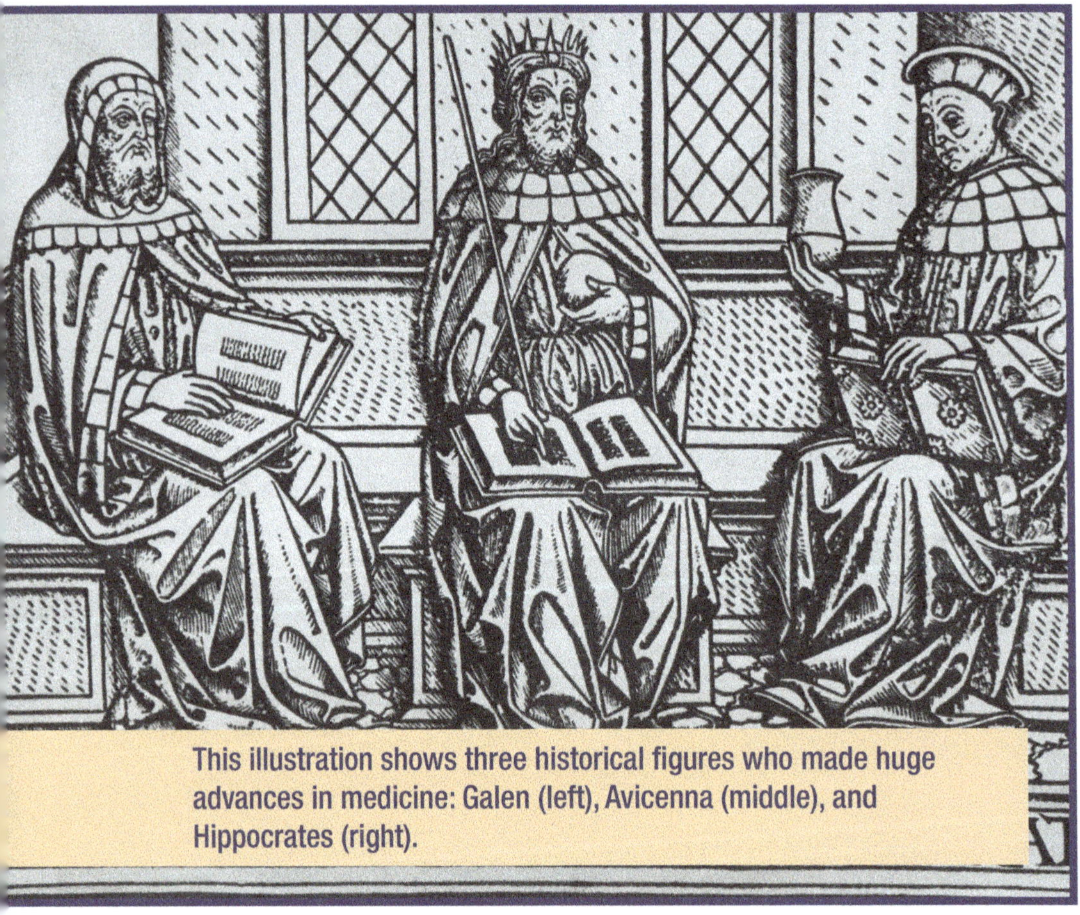

This illustration shows three historical figures who made huge advances in medicine: Galen (left), Avicenna (middle), and Hippocrates (right).

MANY NAMES, ONE STI

Some people don't know gonorrhea by its real name. That's because it has a lot of nicknames; it's also known as GC, the dose, the drop, and most commonly, the clap. But what does "the clap" even mean?

We don't know the true origin or reason behind this nickname, but there are several theories. Some people think it comes from the French word *clapier*, which means brothel. Since many cases of gonorrhea came from brothels, this name seems fitting. However, other people trace the word back to an Old English term, "clappen," which means to throb (which happens with inflammation). Another theory states that the nickname came from a rough (and fortunately outdated) medical treatment of clapping an infected penis against a hard surface with a big, hardback book in order to remove pus. Another theory says "the clap" comes from a clapping sensation that an infected person feels during urination. Regardless, gonorrhea by any other name is still a very painful infection.

Gonorrhea wasn't only a private issue in history; it also became political. By 1161, the English Parliament had enacted a law to halt the spread of gonorrhea; they referred to the condition as "the perilous infirmity of burning." Gonorrhea was often linked with war, conquest, and migration. Some sources indicate that Roman soldiers who fought alongside Julius Caesar (100–40 BCE) had gonorrhea. During the Crimean War of 1853–1856 (a conflict that pitted Russia against France, Britain, the Ottoman Empire, and Sardinia), illnesses—including STIs like gonorrhea—killed more people than combat. Towns and ports where soldiers landed often had a high rate of infection because of sexual activity.

The American Civil War saw around 100,000 documented cases of gonorrhea. Gonorrhea was also an issue with United States soldiers in both world wars. During World War I (1914–1918), the U.S. Army discharged more than 10,000 soldiers due to STIs. Only the devastating flu pandemic of 1918–1919 resulted

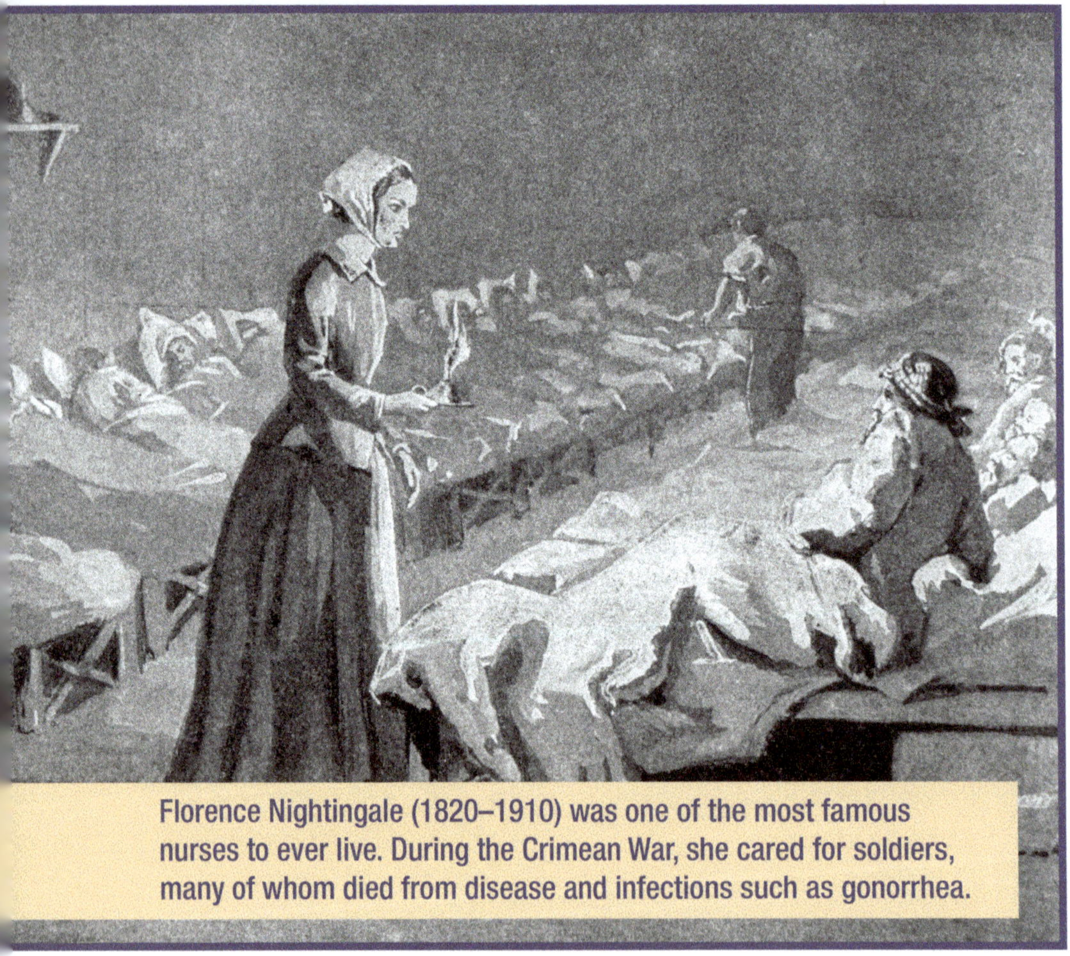

Florence Nightingale (1820–1910) was one of the most famous nurses to ever live. During the Crimean War, she cared for soldiers, many of whom died from disease and infections such as gonorrhea.

in more lost duty days than STIs during the war. The American War Department also ordered that any soldier who didn't get treatment for their STI would be tried and imprisoned. While French and British armies gave out condoms to their soldiers, the U.S. Army would do no such thing—and instead preached abstinence. During World War II (1939–1945), posters were used to warn soldiers about the danger of spending time with prostitutes. Posters reminded the men, "You can't beat the Axis if you get VD [venereal disease]" and "Fool the Axis—Use Prophylaxis [protection]." Military men were lectured and shown movies about the dangers of getting an STI from prostitutes. Condoms were doled out daily—a shift from the U.S. military's thinking during World War I. Gonorrhea was also widespread among U.S. soldiers fighting in the Korean War (1950–1953) and the Vietnam War (1965–1975).

DISCOVERING BAD BACTERIA

Before microscopes, the discovery of bacteria, and modern medicine, STIs like gonorrhea were a mystery. What caused them? And how could they effectively be treated? Albert Ludwig Sigesmund Neisser (1855–1916), a German venereologist, was the first person to identify the bacteria responsible for gonorrhea—*Neisseria gonorrhoeae*. In 1879, 24-year-old Neisser published his first paper, which explained how he had identified what he called "micro-cocci" in the samples taken from 34 subjects. He further explained how they specifically resulted in gonorrhea.

Neisser made important contributions in the field

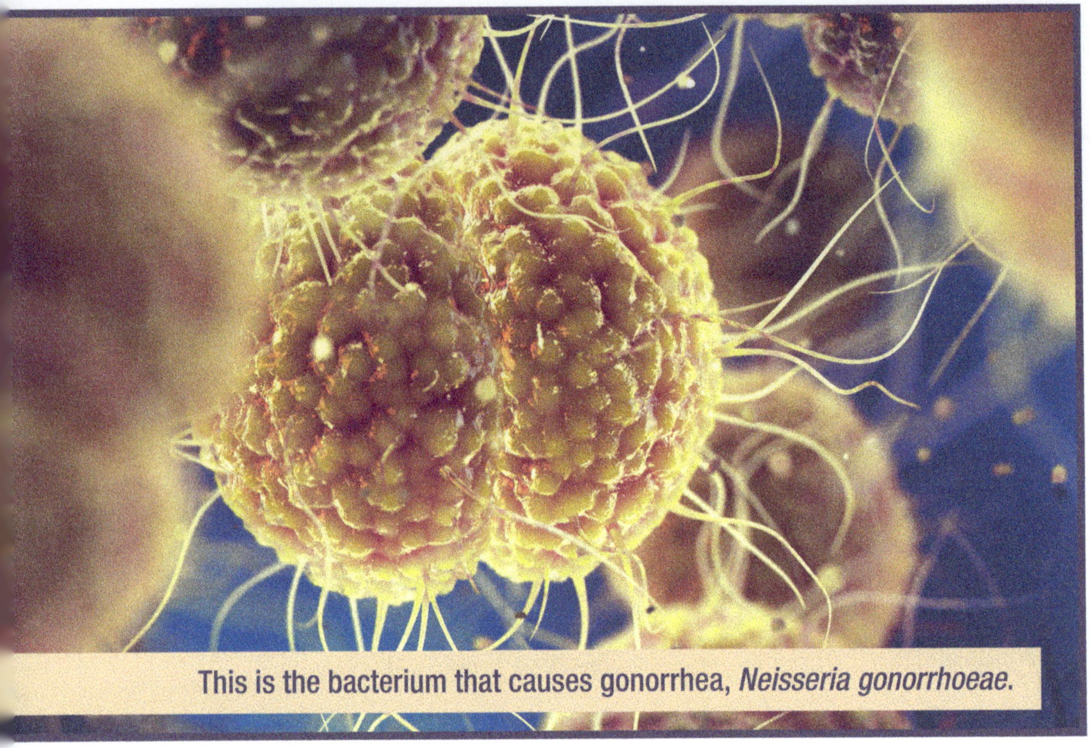

This is the bacterium that causes gonorrhea, *Neisseria gonorrhoeae*.

of venereology—the study of sexually transmitted infections—through his work on gonorrhea and later, syphilis. He dedicated his life to advocating for public health and the prevention of STIs. Neisser spoke out against the prevailing attitude that prostitutes were to be blamed for the spread of gonorrhea. In addition, he worked to educate the public about STIs and urged health agencies to make educating the public a priority. His experiments provided insight into STIs but sometimes had a serious cost. For example, he experimented with syphilis transmission in apes and monkeys, as well as other animals. He also injected four young prostitutes with a serum derived from patients with syphilis, which angered many people.

TREATMENTS OVER TIME

Treatments for gonorrhea have greatly improved over time. In fact, many treatments before the 20th century only made the condition worse. Without proper treatments, people could have serious complications like pelvic inflammatory disease, infertility, and even death. Early treatments for gonorrhea included injecting mercury into the urethra, flushing the urethra with very hot water, and putting very hot instruments on the genitals. Physicians also used silver-based treatments from the 19th century until the mid-20th century. Some put patients into "fever cabinets," which looked like tanning beds. Patients had to endure the heat for hours, thinking it would burn the infection from them. These ineffective and even harmful treatments were fortunately replaced by antibiotics.

In 1940s, antibiotics were introduced as an effective cure for gonorrhea. At last, something helped. In fact, the antibiotics did such a good job that some people thought gonorrhea was soon going to be eradicated, or wiped out. Dr. John Mahoney from the U.S Public Health Service wrote in 1949, "As a result of antibiotic therapy, gonorrhea has almost passed from the scene as an important clinical and public entity."

Unfortunately, Dr. Mahoney and other medical professionals did not anticipate the gonorrhea bacterium's ability to adapt and thrive. It quickly became resistant to the initial type of antibiotics, and different antibiotics had to be used. This is a problem that has only grown. In the CDC's 2013 and 2019 Antibiotic Resistance Threats Report, the agency classified antibiotic-resistant gonorrhea an "urgent threat." That's because bacteria are developing resistance to antibiotics at a faster rate than new antibiotics can be developed and used. This means doctors can run out of antibiotic options for their patients with gonorrhea.

The future of gonorrhea treatments may include a vaccine. One study out of New Zealand found that the vaccine for another infection—meningitis—may protect people from gonorrhea. That's because the bacteria that cause meningitis and gonorrhea are similar. A vaccine to protect against gonorrhea may be just a few

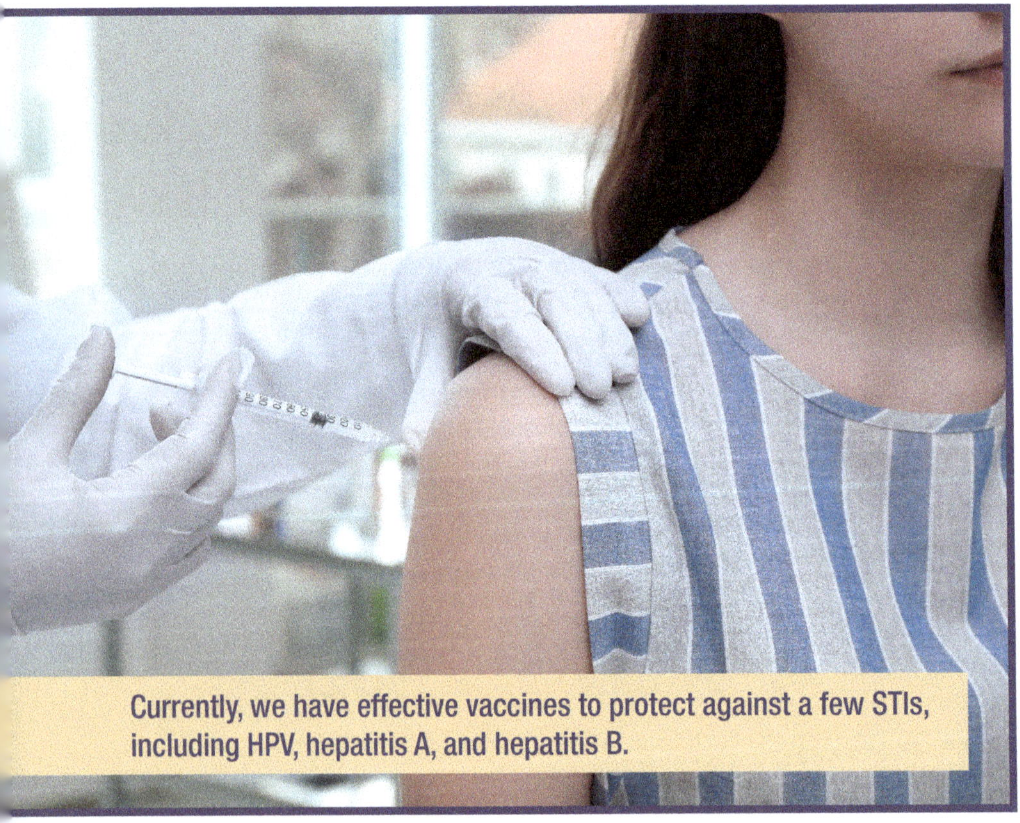

Currently, we have effective vaccines to protect against a few STIs, including HPV, hepatitis A, and hepatitis B.

years away from use. Until a vaccine can be developed, however, preventing the spread of gonorrhea is the best way to keep people safe from its effects.

MYTHS AND FACTS

MYTH

Condoms will only protect you from STIs when used during vaginal sex.

FACT

Condoms can protect you from STIs when used during anal sex, oral sex, and vaginal sex.

MYTH

You can give someone gonorrhea from using a shared toilet seat.

FACT

Gonorrhea can only be transmitted through contact with the genitals, such as through anal, oral, or vaginal sex. It can sometimes be transmitted from mother to baby during birth.

MYTH

If someone has gonorrhea, they will have obvious symptoms.

FACT

Many people who have gonorrhea aren't symptomatic. Biological females are less likely to have symptoms than biological males.

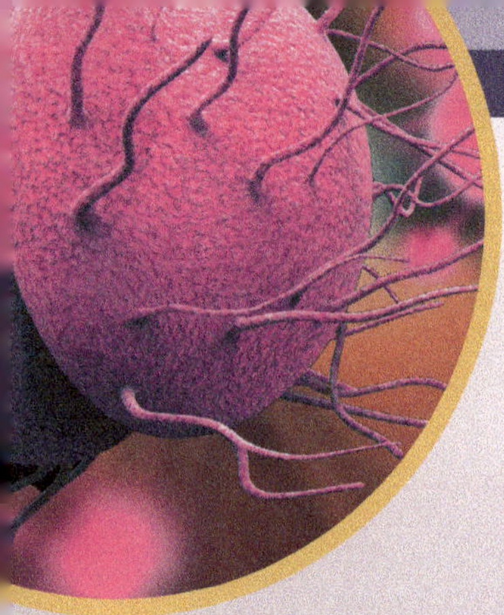

CHAPTER 2

SEX, SIGNS, AND SYMPTOMS

You might worry that you can contract gonorrhea from a toilet seat. You might worry you can get it from kissing someone who has it. However, the overwhelming majority of cases stem from sex. Learning about what kind of sexual behaviors can pass on STIs like gonorrhea can help keep you safe.

LET'S TALK ABOUT SEX

Imagine that you or your sexual partner have tested positive for gonorrhea, but the other person is negative. How could one person spread it to another? Anal, oral, and vaginal sex all spread gonorrhea from one

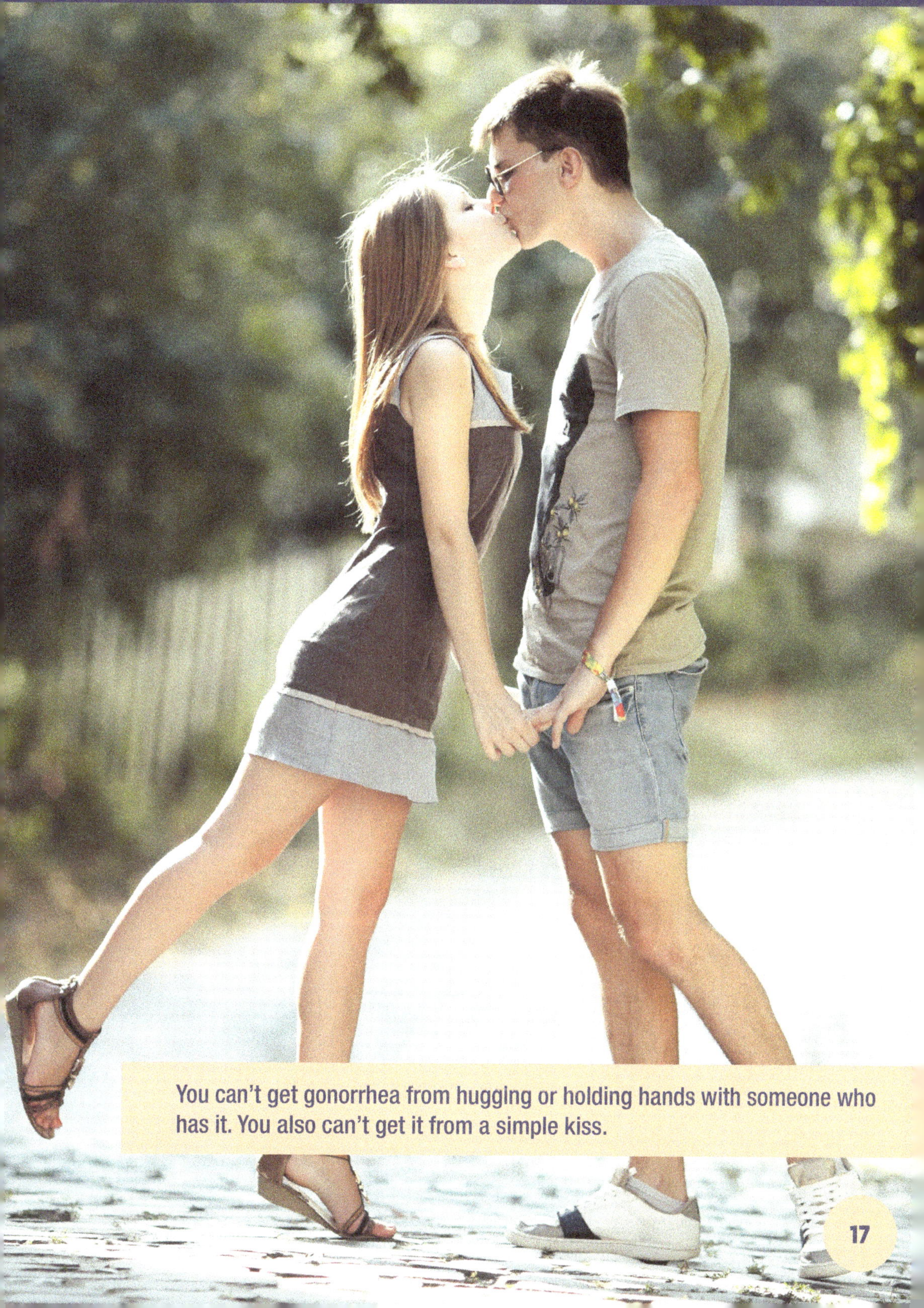

You can't get gonorrhea from hugging or holding hands with someone who has it. You also can't get it from a simple kiss.

infected person to their sexual partner. It doesn't matter if the couple is in a heterosexual (opposite sex) or homosexual (same sex) relationship. Any type of sex is a risk between an infected person and another person. Also, a biological male does not have to ejaculate to pass on the infection.

Because the bacterium is found in the semen and vaginal fluids, this means the disease can also be transmitted by sharing sexual toys that have not been cleaned. When infected body fluids come into contact with the body's mucous membranes, the bacterium thrives in the warm, moist reproductive tract. It settles in and begins to spread through a biological female's cervix, uterus, and fallopian tubes or a biological male's urethra. For those engaging in anal and oral sex, the bacteria may spread through the anus or the mouth and throat.

Anyone who has sex with an infected person is susceptible to getting gonorrhea, but some people are at a higher risk than others. These include people who have had gonorrhea in the past. It also includes people who have had other STIs in the past, those with multiple sexual partners, and people who are sex workers. But people with multiple partners aren't the only people who contract gonorrhea—it only takes one time and one partner to get it.

SIGNS AND SYMPTOMS

How does gonorrhea show up in the body? How can you tell if what you're experiencing is gonorrhea, or something else? To officially diagnose you, doctors will need to take a sample. However, there are some symptoms that can signal that you might have gonorrhea.

Gonorrhea is an infection that sometimes causes symptoms, and sometimes does not. If you have an infection or other illness and don't have symptoms, you are asymptomatic. That is one of the biggest problems with STIs like gonorrhea. If people don't feel the symptoms, they assume they don't have it. Then they don't take precautions to stop the spread and end up passing it on. Approximately four out of five females and one out of ten males who get gonorrhea either have no symptoms or have mild ones that aren't noticeable. Many women may notice the symptoms but assume they have a yeast infection and treat it with topical medication. People might assume their fever and discomfort is nothing more than a case of the flu.

If you are sexually active, it's very important that you pay close attention to possible symptoms. Symptoms typically begin one to fourteen days after sex with an infected partner. In biological males, it is often a matter of a few days, but for biological females, it can take weeks to months for them to appear.

People who are biologically male have certain symptoms that are common with gonorrhea. They may have a discharge from the penis that is white, yellow, or green. This is called dysuria. This means they have an infection in their urethra. They may also have an infection that causes pain in their testicles or scrotum. They may feel as if they need to urinate more frequently.

People who are biologically female experience different symptoms with gonorrhea. They might have

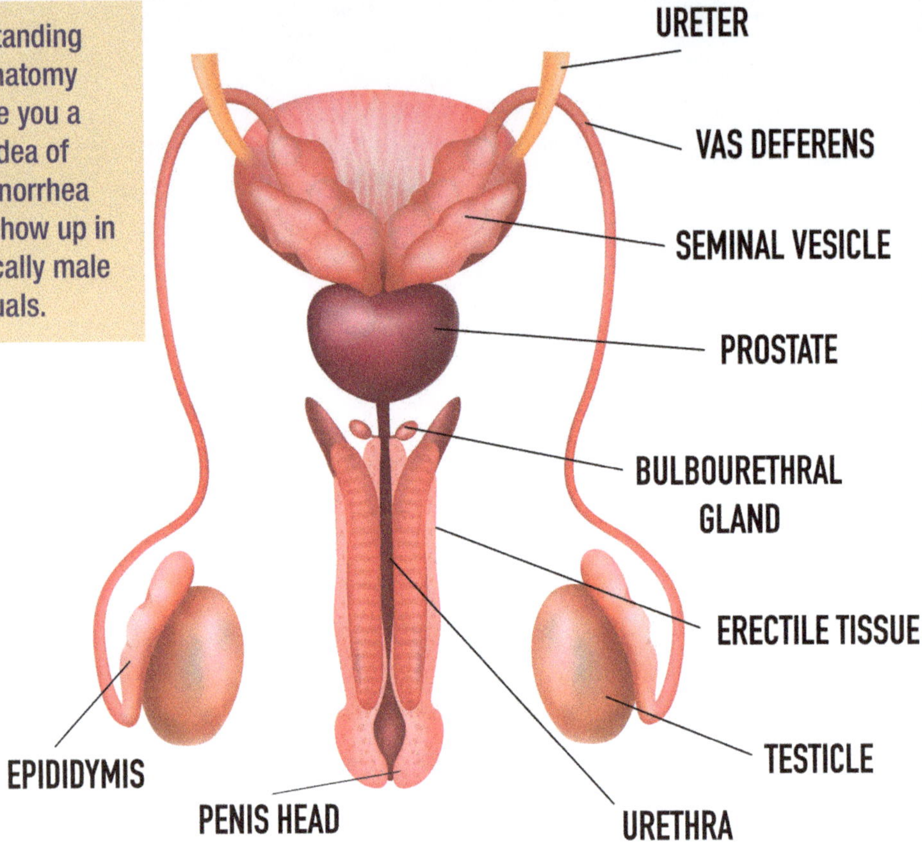

Understanding male anatomy can give you a better idea of how gonorrhea might show up in biologically male individuals.

discharge from the vagina that is yellow, green, or bloody. They may have swelling or tenderness of the vulva. They may also bleed between their periods, experience pain during intercourse or urination, or have abdominal or pelvic pain.

Gonorrhea can often be mistaken for a urinary tract infection (UTI) or vaginal infection in biologically female individuals. That's because many of the same symptoms occur in other infections. For example, a urinary tract infection can cause pain during sex and urination, while a yeast infection can cause discharge from the vagina and swelling of the vulva. This is why it's important to have a doctor or another medical professional diagnose you if you feel symptoms of an STD or another infection of the genitals or urinary tract. It's not always easy to tell them apart by symptoms alone—and often testing a sample is the only way to officially diagnose with certainty.

Regardless of biological sex, people can contract a rectal infection, which may cause itching of the anus, discharge from the anus, and painful bowel movements. They might even get a fever. People can also have a gonorrhea infection that affects their mouth, throat, and eyes. Mouth and throat infections are often asymptomatic, but sometimes include a sore throat, redness in the throat, fever, or swollen lymph nodes in the neck. Although genital gonorrhea can only be passed through sexual activity, there are some studies that suggest that kissing with tongues involved may be able to transmit oral (mouth) gonorrhea. The problem with oral gonorrhea is that it's often asymptomatic or seems like any other throat infection, and people don't get treatment for it.

If you have any symptoms or know that you've had sex with an infected person, it's important to get treatment before complications arise. Complications from untreated gonorrhea can cause serious damage to your body, and even death.

PELVIC INFLAMMATORY DISEASE

Throughout history, STIs could be life-threatening because of the lack of effective treatments. However, with proper treatment, most people today don't have any lasting effects. Complications enter the picture, however, when STIs are left untreated. For biological females, an untreated STI, especially gonorrhea or chlamydia, can result in a far more serious condition called pelvic inflammatory disease, or PID. PID is an infection of a female's reproductive organs. It's caused when the microorganisms from STIs move up from the cervix and vagina to the upper genital tract. PID can result in infertility and can permanently damage the reproductive organs. Statistics show that one out of five females with untreated gonorrhea will develop PID.

The symptoms of PID are often subtle and easy to overlook. The most common symptoms include lower abdominal pain, mild pelvic pain, pelvic organ tenderness, uterine tenderness, pain with intercourse, and cervical tenderness. A biologically female person with PID might also have increased vaginal discharge and irregular periods. Inflammation and fever are also signs of PID.

If PID isn't treated, it can result in scarred fallopian tubes, pelvic adhesions, chronic pelvic pain, ectopic pregnancies, or infertility. While antibiotics can cure PID, they cannot reverse the scarring caused by the infection. That's why it's so important to seek diagnosis and treatment for STIs and PID from the first sign or symptom.

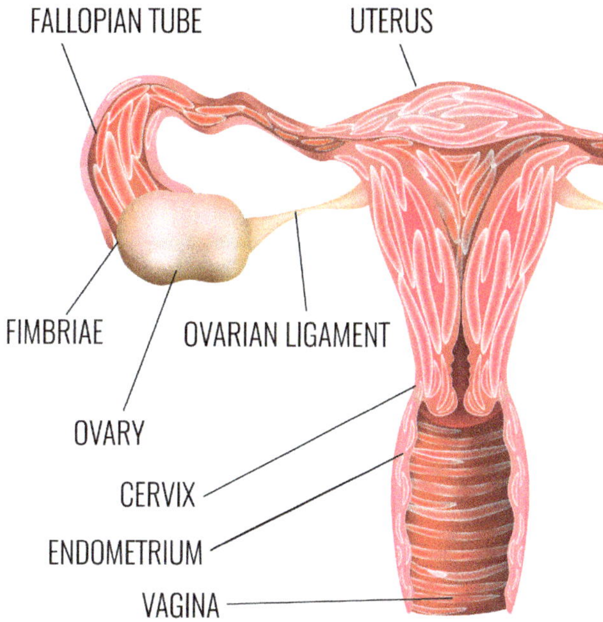

This diagram shows the different parts of the female reproductive system, some of which are at risk with untreated pelvic inflammatory disease (PID).

BABIES AT RISK

Gonorrhea can sometimes have devastating effects on newborn babies. If a pregnant person contracts gonorrhea, the infection can be passed to her baby during labor and delivery. People who get gonorrhea while they are pregnant carry a higher risk of miscarriage. The baby's amniotic sac and the fluid in it can become infected. There is also a high risk for preterm birth, or birth before a baby is fully developed.

Gonorrhea in babies often affects the baby's eyes and can cause blindness if not treated. In most states, all babies are automatically treated with medicated eye drops soon after birth in case the mother has gonorrhea. In rare cases, the infection can also pass to other parts of the baby's body, resulting in blood or joint infections or meningitis, an inflammation of the membranes around the brain and the spinal cord. This makes it even more important for pregnant people to take care of their sexual health and get tested and treated as soon as possible.

SERIOUS COMPLICATIONS

Some people don't take gonorrhea seriously because many people experience only mild symptoms. However, untreated gonorrhea can lead to serious and life-changing complications for both biologically male and female individuals.

For biologically male people, untreated gonorrhea can reduce their fertility, or ability to be a biological father. In some cases, it even makes them sterile, or completely unable to biologically father children. It can also lead to painful inflammation of the testicles or epididymis, as well as urethral scarring. Gonorrhea can also put a person at increased risk of getting or giving HIV, and infection can spread to other parts of the body, including the blood, joints, or heart.

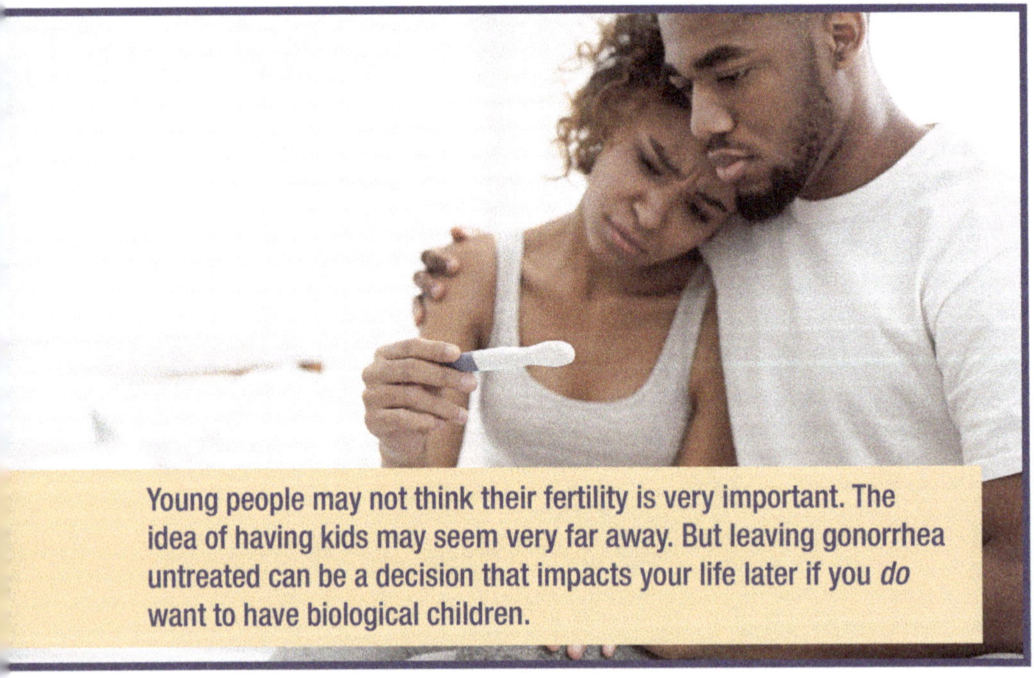

Young people may not think their fertility is very important. The idea of having kids may seem very far away. But leaving gonorrhea untreated can be a decision that impacts your life later if you *do* want to have biological children.

For biologically female individuals, gonorrhea can also impact their ability to start or maintain a pregnancy. They might suffer infertility when they decide to get pregnant, or they might have an ectopic pregnancy. In an ectopic pregnancy, the embryo attaches outside of the uterus and cannot develop but can cause significant pain and blood loss. If a woman contracts gonorrhea while pregnant, it can lead to miscarriage (loss of a fetus before 20 or 28 weeks of pregnancy) or stillbirth (death of a baby before or during delivery). It can also lead to premature labor, or having the baby early. Females who aren't pregnant can also suffer complications such as PID and infections of the blood, joints, and eyes. Infection may spread to other parts of the body, including the blood, joints, or heart. As with males, females with untreated gonorrhea are at increased risk of getting or spreading HIV.

What's the connection between HIV and gonorrhea? HIV, or human immunodeficiency virus, attacks the body's immune system so the body can't fight off infection. If a person living with HIV contracts gonorrhea, the bacterium can cause an increase in the amount of HIV in the genital and rectal fluids of a person with HIV. This increases the chance that a person with HIV would pass HIV on to their sexual partner or partners. Untreated gonorrhea also puts people at an increased risk for contracting HIV. There is currently no cure for HIV, but there is effective treatment. Untreated HIV may develop into AIDS, or acquired immunodeficiency syndrome.

Approximately three out of every 100 people with untreated gonorrhea are at risk of developing disseminated gonococcal infection, or DGI. This condition causes arthritis (joint pain) and skin sores. It can be treated, but if it is not, it can permanently damage the joints of the body. Also called gonococcal arthritis, it is more commonly seen in young, healthy individuals than older people.

Asymptomatic gonorrhea or gonorrhea with mild symptoms can be easy to ignore. You may just want to pretend it's not happening to you. Or you may think you don't need treatment. But it can have serious consequences and complications if left untreated.

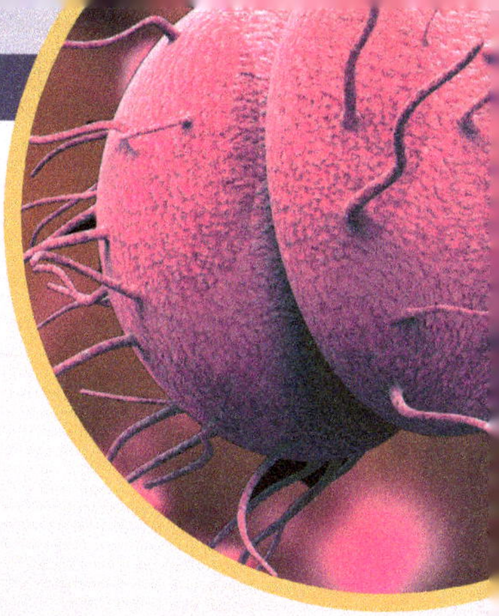

CHAPTER 3

STAYING SMART ABOUT SEX

Gonorrhea may sound pretty scary. As with all STIs, you want to avoid it whenever possible. And fortunately, if you practice safe sexual behaviors, you can significantly lower your risk of contracting an STI.

The only way to be 100 percent safe from an STI is to be abstinent, or not have sex. Many young people choose to be abstinent for many reasons. However, other young people choose to have sex for many different reasons. It's important to know what's right for you, and to make decisions that can keep you safe and well.

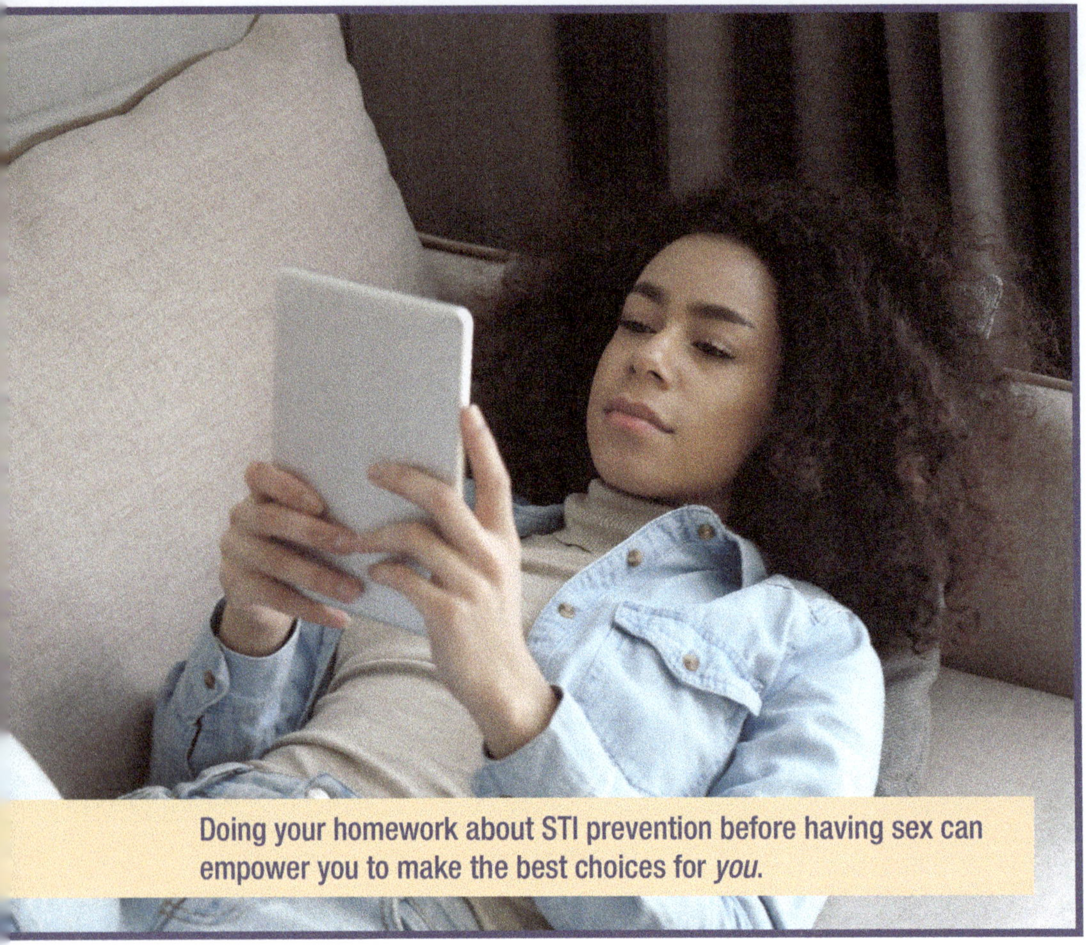

Doing your homework about STI prevention before having sex can empower you to make the best choices for *you*.

In 2019, the CDC reported that of the high school students it surveyed, 38 percent had had sex. However, 46 percent of those students hadn't used a condom the last time they had sex, and less than 10 percent of all students had been tested for STDs that year. Risky sexual behaviors contribute to high rates of HIV, STIs, and pregnancy among young people. If you choose to have sex, you can learn how to stay safe and smart, and take control of your sexual health.

PICKING YOUR PARTNER

Who you have sex with makes a big difference in your risk of contracting an STI. If you are going to be sexually active, you decrease your chances of STIs by having sex with only one partner. Agreeing to do this is referred to as "mutual monogamy." It makes sense that the fewer people involved, the lower your risk of getting an STI. If you're having sex with multiple people, you increase your chances that one of them has an STI. Having a conversation with your partner is a very mature step; you can decide to only have sex with one another and to be open and honest about your sexual history and STI test results. If a person isn't willing to do this, you can reconsider if they are the right person for you to be having sex with.

Sometimes sex isn't between two committed people, though. People may hook up with people they don't know or have casual sex with one or more partners. In that case, it's necessary to get tested regularly and always use protection, such as a condom.

Certain behaviors can impact your sexual decision-making. Drinking alcohol or using drugs lowers inhibitions and makes it more likely you will end up having unprotected or unintentional sex. Under the influence of alcohol or drugs, you might make decisions you wouldn't normally make. This can make it harder to make smart sexual decisions about who you're going to have sex with.

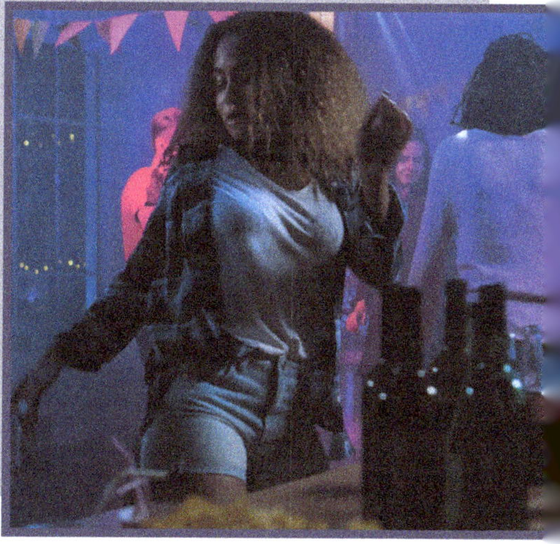

Alcohol and drugs can impair your judgment and make you less likely to make safe choices.

Some people are forced into sex, either by someone they know or someone they don't know. The CDC found this was true for 7 percent of high school students they surveyed, and that's only what was reported. The numbers are likely higher. If someone forces you to have sex, it's important to know that it's not your fault and you're not alone. You can still do what's best for your health and wellness by getting support, getting tested, and getting the treatment you need.

COMMUNICATION IS KEY

Communication is one of the most important parts of a healthy relationship. If someone isn't willing to communicate with you about their sexual history or STI status, they may not be a smart choice as a sexual partner.

Before you have sex with someone, find out if they have ever had any kind of STI or have been tested recently. Find out if your partner has had a lot of sexual partners before you. This is important to know. Unless both of you have been completely abstinent up until now, it's best that you both get tested. Also make sure your partner is as educated as you are about STIs and how to prevent them. Remember that vaginal, oral, and anal sex all have high risk factors, so whatever the two of you do needs to be discussed. Some people aren't very nervous about contracting STIs and might be unwilling to hear the facts. It's important that you educate others when you can and stand your ground if something makes you uncomfortable or doesn't feel safe.

Some people feel embarrassed to talk about sex, contraception, and STIs with their partner. But just remember how important the topic is for both of you to remain healthy. Approach STIs as a medical issue. You'd want to know if your partner had mono before you kissed because you don't want to get it, right? It's the same thing with an STI. Next, prepare what you are going to say before you start. What's important to you? What are you concerned about?

Make sure to choose a good time and place to talk. In between classes in the hallway is not a good choice.

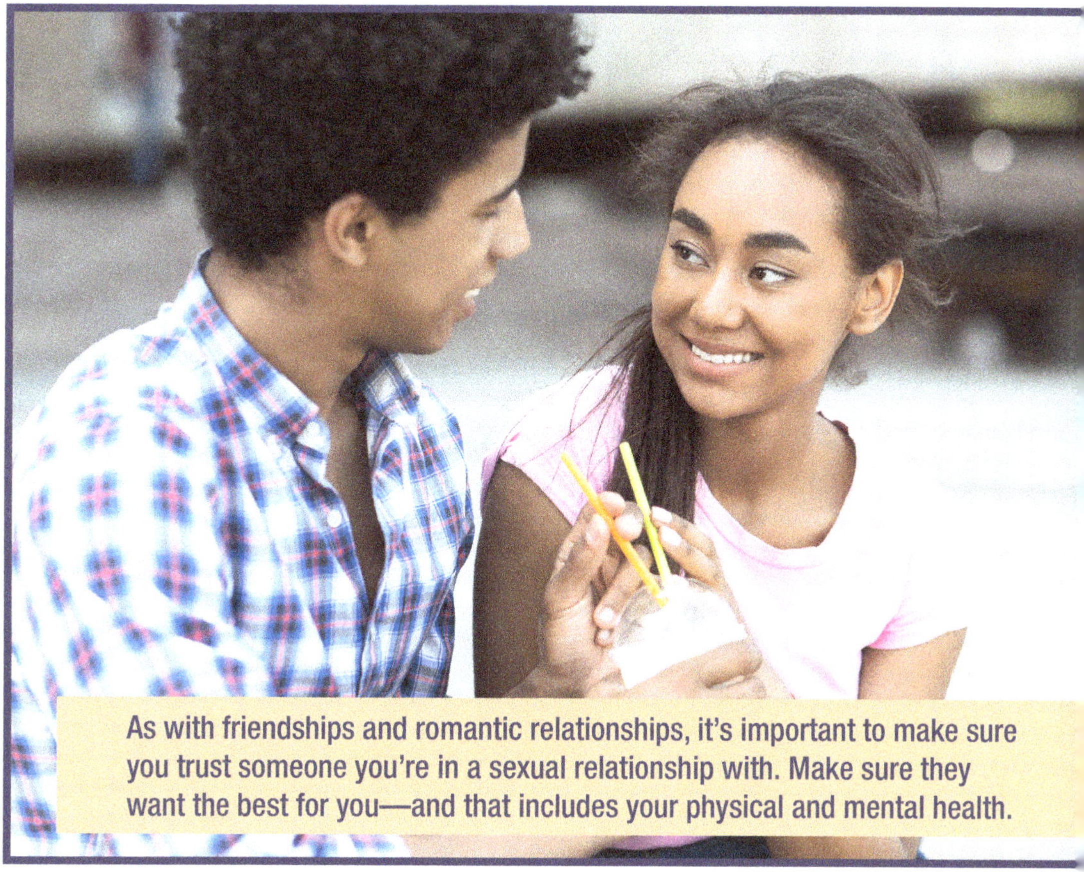

As with friendships and romantic relationships, it's important to make sure you trust someone you're in a sexual relationship with. Make sure they want the best for you—and that includes your physical and mental health.

You need a quiet, private place to be together and talk honestly. Don't wait until you're already starting to have sex either. You want to choose a time when you are both thinking clearly and not in a rush.

THE BEST PROTECTION

Protecting against STIs and protecting against pregnancy are both essential parts of taking responsibility for your sexual health. There are a number of choices that protect against both STIs and pregnancy, including female condoms (internal condoms) and male condoms (external condoms). Dental dams also protect against STIs during oral sex.

A dental dam is a small, thin, square piece of latex that is used during oral-vaginal or oral-anal sex. It's important to remember that STIs can be spread through oral sex, and dental dams are your best protection in that case. They prevent STIs by keeping vaginal and anal fluids away from the mouth. Dams are frequently used with water-based lubricants, and like regular condoms, they are for one-time use only. They can be purchased online, but some clinics like Planned Parenthood and college student health services may offer them for free. Dental dams can also be made from regular condoms by cutting off the tip and cutting down one side.

While female condoms aren't considered quite as effective at preventing STIs as the male condom, they are still recommended. A female condom is a pouch that is inserted into the vagina. It is made out of strong plastic called polyurethane or a substance called nitrile.

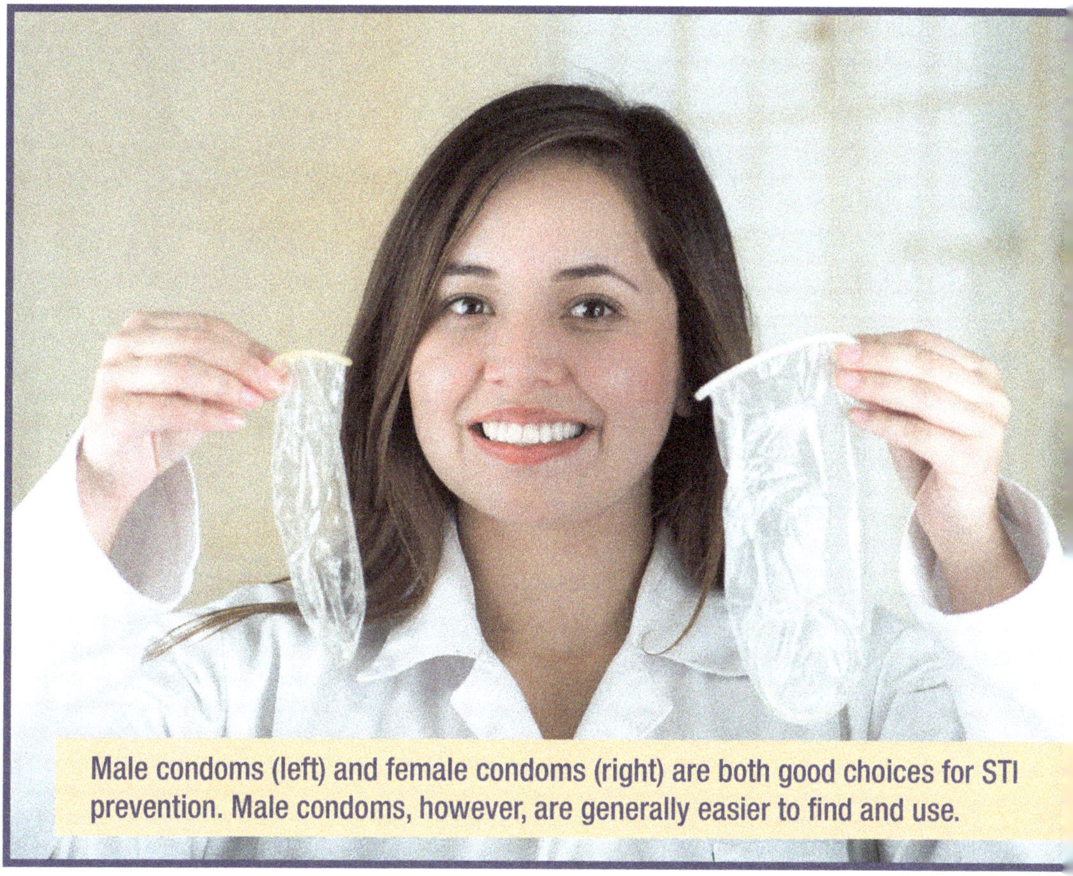

Male condoms (left) and female condoms (right) are both good choices for STI prevention. Male condoms, however, are generally easier to find and use.

It has flexible rings on each end. The ring at the closed end holds the pouch in place. The ring at the open end remains outside the vaginal opening during sex. For anal intercourse, the pouch is inserted into the anus.

Like male condoms, female condoms are generally found in drugstores and do not require a prescription. They can be used with oil- or water-based lubricants as well. They can be used during menstruation or pregnancy, and they can be inserted up to eight hours before sex. They should not be used, however, in conjunction with a male condom as the two can rub together and cause discomfort or breakage.

Male condoms have been the main way to prevent STIs for decades. According to the CDC, both laboratory and epidemiologic studies have shown that latex condoms provide a truly effective barrier against even the tiniest STI pathogens. Of course, their effectiveness relies completely on consistent and correct use, and users are encouraged to check condoms for holes or tears and to use a condom throughout the entire sex act, from initial sexual contact to ejaculation. Also, condoms should never be reused.

Male condoms are usually made out of latex (hence the nickname "rubbers") or polyurethane. They vary in color, size, and amount of lubrication and spermicide. Rolled over the erect penis, the condom prevents direct contact between the penis and vagina or rectum, so there is far less risk of contracting an STI. As every study has shown, using condoms is very effective for preventing infection. Using them properly is important, so make sure both you and your partner are educated about how to do it right.

Even if you have taken every precaution, it's still good to get tested regularly if you have sex with someone who has had other partners. You can get tested through your doctor or a sexual health clinic like Planned Parenthood. That will give you peace of mind and the ability to treat any infection quickly.

CONDOMS FOR THE WIN!

According to Planned Parenthood, the earliest known illustration of a biologically male person using a condom during sex dates from 12,000 to 15,000 years ago. The illustration was found painted on a cave wall in what is today France. Condoms have been used since the 16th century to protect people from contracting STIs and since the 18th century to keep people from getting pregnant. They are also incredibly effective in both regards, and today's condoms are designed to be more effective than ever.

Many studies have looked at how effective male condoms are when it comes to preventing STIs. A 2005 study surveyed 509 biologically female teens and found that consistent and correct use of condoms gave "significant protection" against gonorrhea. It actually found that none of the subjects of the study contracted gonorrhea if they and their partner or partners used condoms consistently and correctly. But sometimes people stop using condoms, either because they are expensive or unavailable, or for other personal reasons. A 2017 study (Margo Mullinax et. al.) looked at why people discontinue condoms. The study's authors wrote: "Condoms remain the best form of simultaneous protection against sexually transmitted infections (STIs) and unintended pregnancies, both of which remain persistent sexual health concerns among emerging adults." The United Nations Joint Programme on HIV/AIDS, Centers for Disease Control and Prevention, and the World Health Organization also promote the use of male condoms to protect against STIs.

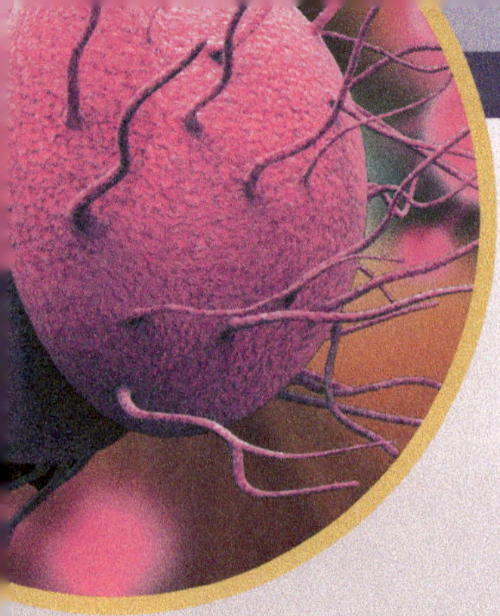

CHAPTER 4

TESTS AND TREATMENT

If you think you've had sex with someone infected with gonorrhea, or if you have symptoms of gonorrhea, it's important that you get tested and treated as soon as possible. Tests are quick and easy, and treatment is often pretty straightforward if the infection is caught quickly enough.

Some people decide not to get tested because they don't feel any symptoms or believe that symptoms will go away. Others don't want a diagnosis because that means they'd have to tell sexual partners that they've been infected. Some people just don't know how to get a test or find treatment. No matter the reason someone might have against testing and treatment, taking care of their sexual health is the best thing they can do for themselves and their partners.

TAKING THE TEST

You might not know where to go for a gonorrhea test. You can search online for the closest testing place near you. Your doctor can give you a test. You can also go to a community health clinic or your local Planned Parenthood health center. You have to be honest with your doctor, nurse, or medical professionals in a clinic so they can best help you. You might be nervous to tell your pediatrician that you've had sex, but they are only there to help, and will want to give you the treatment you need to feel better.

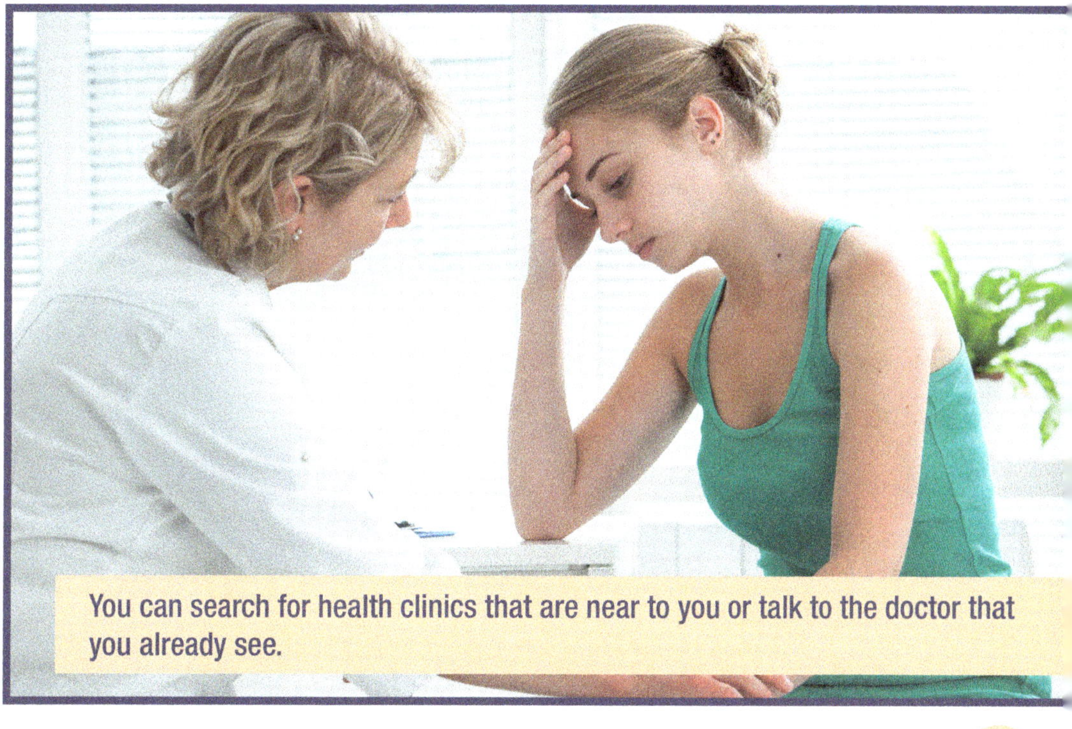

You can search for health clinics that are near to you or talk to the doctor that you already see.

Three types of tests are used to check for gonorrhea: swab, urine, and gram stain. In the swab test, as the name indicates, a swab is taken of the urethra in males or cervix in females. In the past, that is where the testing sites would have stopped. However, today, swabs are also often taken in the throat (for those who have had oral sex), the eye, and the rectum (for those who have had anal sex). Swab samples are sent to a lab where cultures—tests that place the sample in prepared nutrients—are done to see what type of bacteria grow. These tests not only determine if there are any other STIs present but also can help pinpoint which antibiotics will treat the condition best. You should have your results in two to three days.

The gram stain test also takes a swab of the urethra or the cervix, and then the sample is stained with a specific dye that makes the *Neisseria gonorrhoeae* bacteria easy to spot under a microscope. This is the fastest test, but it is not considered as accurate, and many doctor's offices do not have the equipment with which to perform the test. The urine test requires a urine sample to analyze. It tends to be the most expensive of the tests, but it is very accurate and results are usually available the same day.

People who are sexually active should consider getting tested regularly. The CDC recommends that all adults and adolescents between 13 and 64 years old should be tested at least once for HIV. Sexually active, biologically female individuals under 25 years old should be tested for gonorrhea and chlamydia every year. If a female over 25 years old has new or multiple sex partners or a partner with an STD, they should

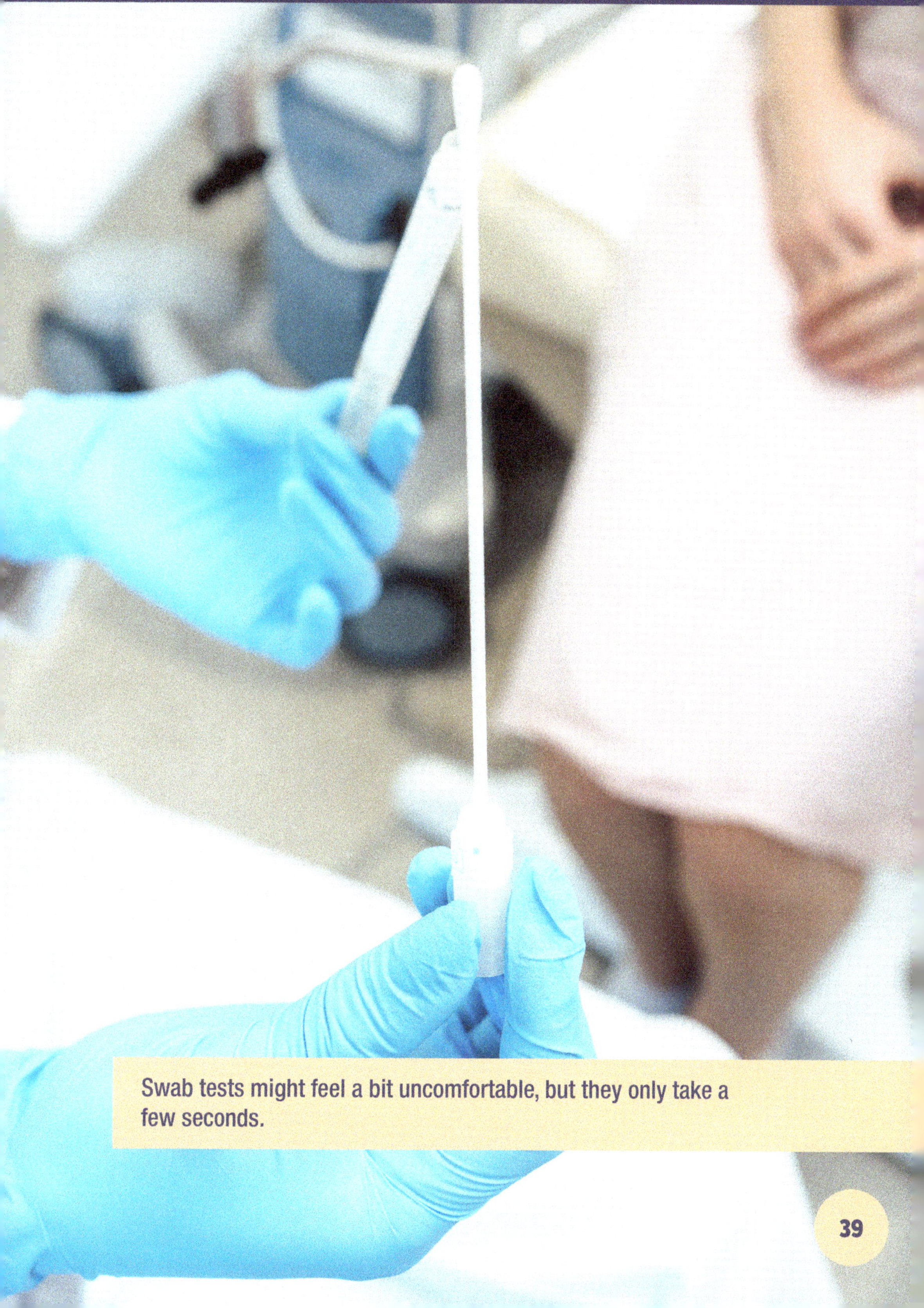

Swab tests might feel a bit uncomfortable, but they only take a few seconds.

be tested each year. People who are pregnant should also be tested for chlamydia and gonorrhea in early pregnancy. Biological males who have sex with other biological males should also be tested at least once a year for gonorrhea.

In recent years, home tests for gonorrhea have become available via the internet. For males, it is usually as simple as sending in a urine sample to be tested in the company's lab. For women, the tests usually require a swab. Companies provide prepaid envelopes for sending in the samples, and results arrive in the mail in two to ten days. This can be a good option for someone who is unable or unwilling to go to a medical professional's office or clinic for testing.

SO, IT'S POSITIVE

Getting a positive test for gonorrhea can bring up a lot of emotions and concerns. You might be anxious about your health. You might be worried to tell your sexual partner. You might be sad or upset. You might even be angry with a sexual partner who gave you the infection. Dealing with these emotions can be difficult, but you also have to take the steps to treat your infection.

Remember, gonorrhea is a common disease, and it is completely curable. The first thing you need to do is get treatment. Talking to your parents or a trusted adult is a good idea. They can help make sure you get to the doctor and get proper medical care. Many parents also love you and are likely to support you in making the best decisions.

Talking to an adult or medical professional about

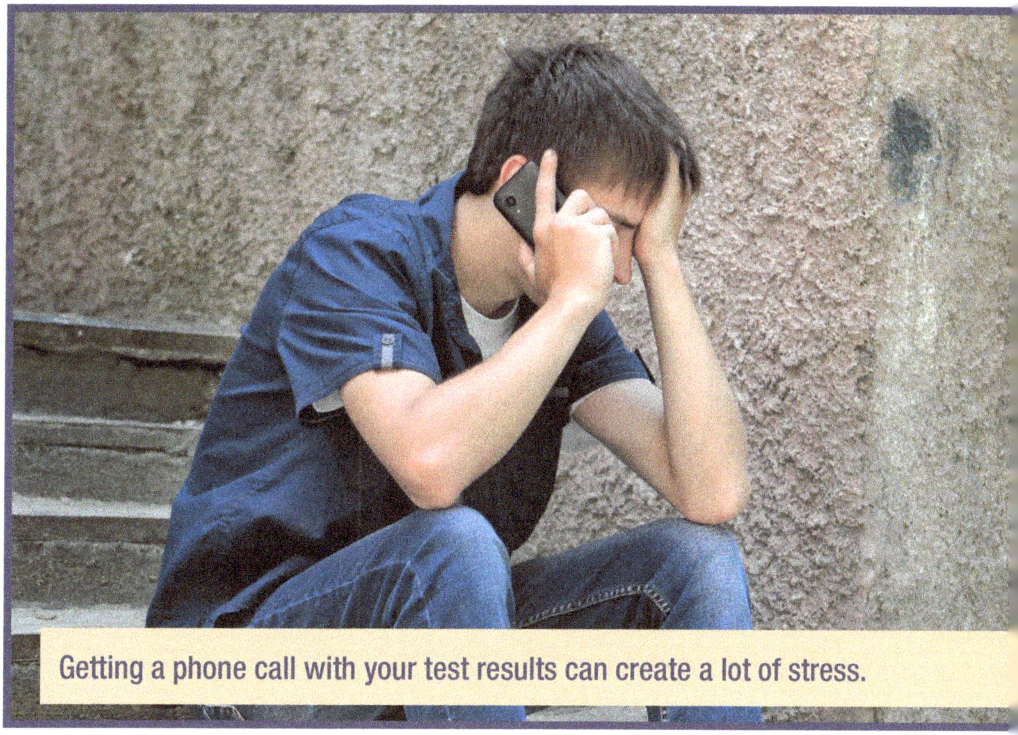

Getting a phone call with your test results can create a lot of stress.

your diagnosis is only one of the conversations you need to have. It is absolutely essential (and the right thing to do) to inform any of the anal, vaginal, or oral sex partners with whom you have had sex within 60 days of the first onset of symptoms and/or positive diagnosis. They deserve to know so that they, too, can get to the doctor and get checked and treated, if necessary. Your health-care provider may help you make a list of sexual partners you've had and come up with a plan for how to tell them.

Telling your partner that you have gonorrhea can feel even more awkward than having the STI conversation about whether they've has been tested and how many partners they've had previously. The rules for how to start this conversation are almost the same, however. Pick a time and place where you can have privacy. Have your information lined up and ready, and don't make the announcement while you're already in the middle of sex. Practice what you're going to say, explain what you have learned about treatment, and then listen patiently in return. Your partner may have a lot of emotions around this news too. Having good communication with one another before a crisis can help you deal with situations like this as a team.

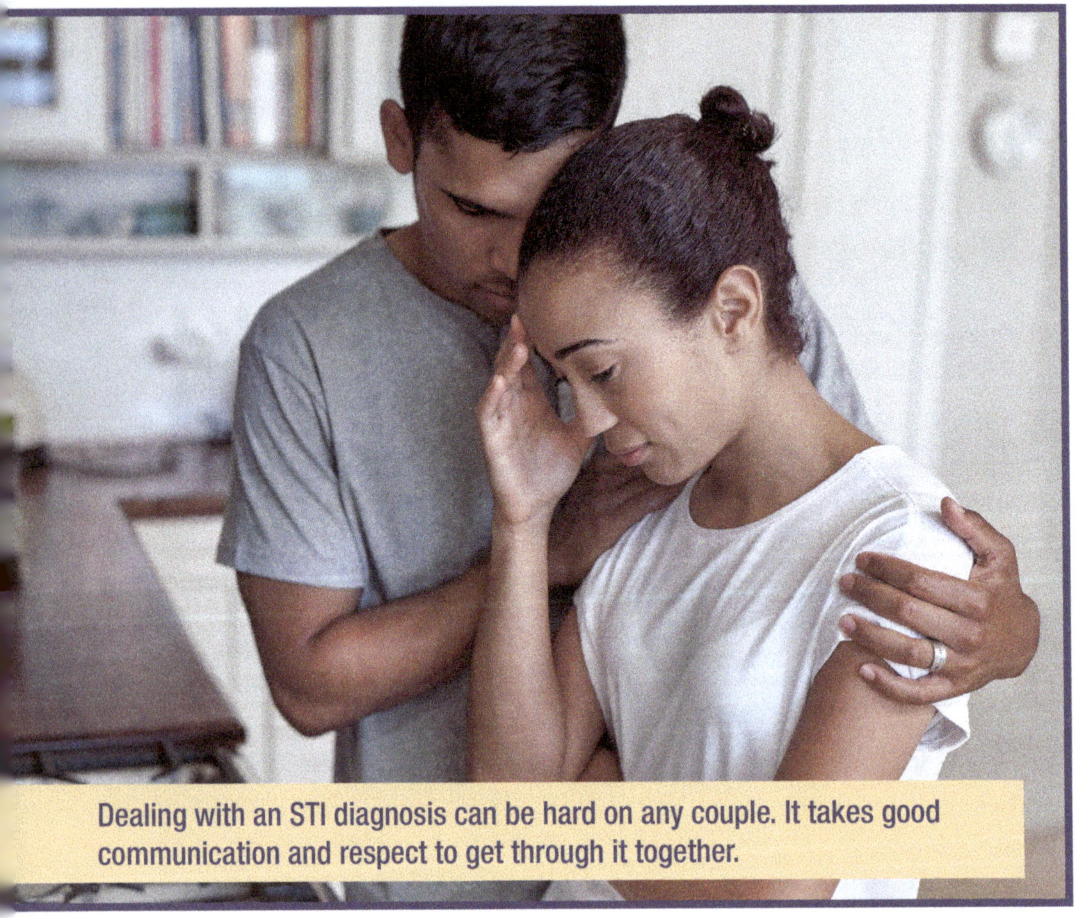

Dealing with an STI diagnosis can be hard on any couple. It takes good communication and respect to get through it together.

ANALYZING THE NUMBERS

If you're diagnosed with gonorrhea, you'll have to tell sexual partners that you're positive. And your doctor or any other medical professional who is treating you will have to tell the CDC. That's because certain diseases are considered to be of significant importance to the general public's health. These diseases must be reported by law to the CDC by the health care provider either via a written report or a telephone call. The list of diseases is long and includes everything from COVID-19 and hepatitis to rabies and yellow fever. STIs, including gonorrhea, are also on this list.

According to the National Institutes of Health, getting these numbers helps researchers identify disease trends. It also helps researchers track disease outbreaks. This can help them make a strategy for dealing with the outbreaks and preventing them from happening or from getting worse. In the case of STIs, the county or state may also try to locate sexual contacts of infected people to ensure they are disease-free or get the treatment they need if already infected. It may feel like an invasion of your privacy to have your STI reported, but these numbers can help keep your community safe.

ANTIBIOTICS TO THE RESCUE

The development and use of antibiotics changed the way gonorrhea was treated. They replaced treatments like flushing the urethra with hot water and injecting harmful chemicals into the genitals, which didn't really help and were very painful.

The type of antibiotics doctors use has changed a number of times over the years. The first was sulfonamide in the 1930s and 1940s, followed by penicillin, tetracycline, spectinomycin, and then ceftriaxone. The type of antibiotic keeps changing because *Neisseria gonorrhoeae* is a relatively smart bacterium. It is clever, with an amazing memory and an ability to resist every antibiotic treatment that is thrown at it. That's why recommendations for treatment of gonorrhea have changed over the years. Currently, the CDC recommends a combination of antibiotics to make sure they are effective. First, an injection of ceftriaxone is given, followed by either a single dose, by pill, of azithromycin or seven days of the drug doxycycline, which is also taken orally. However, some cases of gonorrhea clear up after only one antibiotic in pill form, or pills for seven days.

The rule with antibiotics is that you must take all of them, even if your symptoms have completely

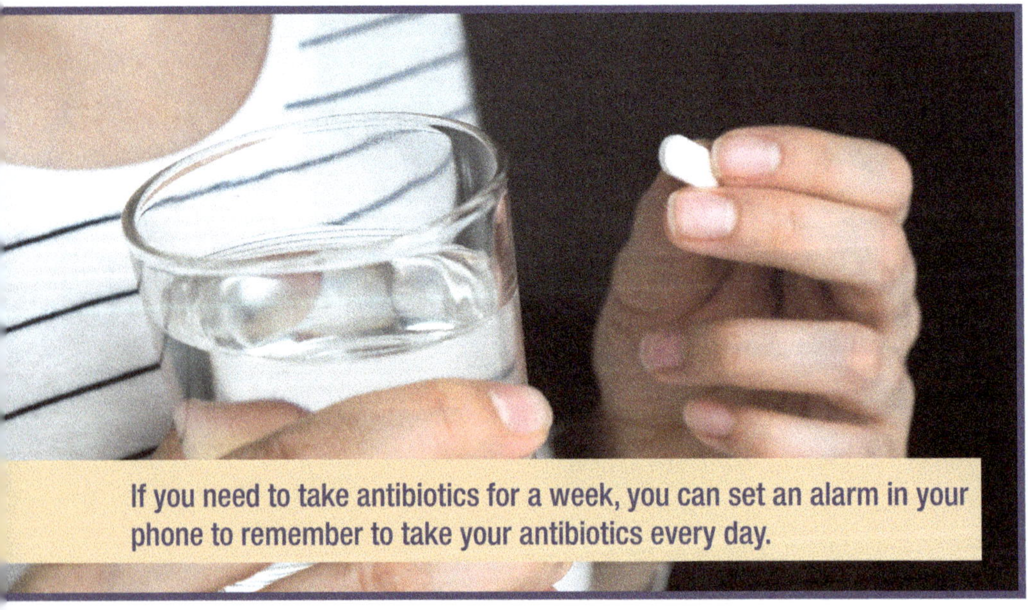

If you need to take antibiotics for a week, you can set an alarm in your phone to remember to take your antibiotics every day.

disappeared before you finish taking the full dose. Also, you should never share your antibiotics with another person, or take antibiotics that were prescribed to someone else. Never take an antibiotic that was prescribed for a previous infection. With correct use, the antibiotics you are prescribed should cure your infection. However, antibiotics can't repair any damage that the infection might have caused, which is why it's important to get treated before you develop complications. While you're recovering, it's smart to avoid having any type of sex with a partner until you have completed your treatment and no longer have any symptoms.

One big problem in the treatment of gonorrhea and other infections is antibiotic resistance. When doctors over-prescribe antibiotics or people overuse them or misuse them, bacteria are more likely to adapt to that antibiotic and make it less effective. It's important for you to go back to your medical provider for further testing if the antibiotic you were given hasn't cleared up your infection. You might be one of those people who have a very resistant strain of gonorrhea, and your doctor not only has to know that but needs to report it as a "treatment failure." You will most likely need a different type of antibiotic. Eventually, new drugs and treatments for gonorrhea will have to be developed to treat antibiotic-resistant cases, but these treatments may be more expensive.

A positive test for gonorrhea is nothing to ignore, but neither is it a reason to panic. Treatments are available—and they are effective. In time, you will be cured of gonorrhea and able to live normally.

10 GREAT QUESTIONS TO ASK A DOCTOR

1. If I don't have any symptoms, could I still give gonorrhea to my partner?
2. How long will my treatment last?
3. What treatments can you provide for the complications of gonorrhea?
4. What happens if this antibiotic doesn't work?
5. What precautions should I take if I do have sex after this diagnosis?
6. Should my sexual partner or partners also be tested?
7. Do I need any other tests after my treatment?
8. Are you testing me for other STIs as well?
9. How can I prevent gonorrhea in the future?
10. What are the side effects of the treatment you are prescribing?

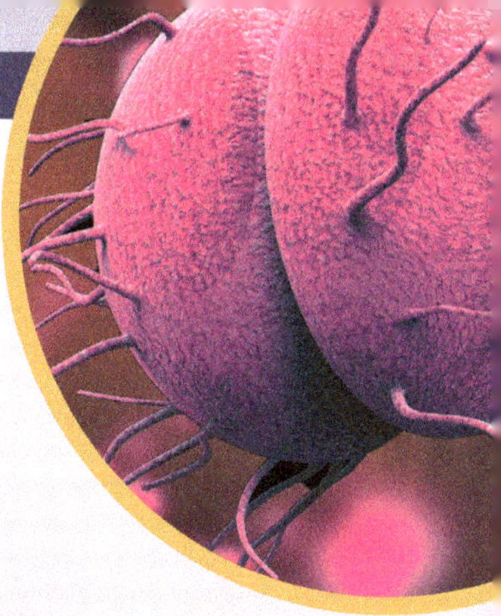

CHAPTER 5

GETTING REAL ABOUT GONORRHEA

Many people suffer from STIs out of shame. There's a stigma around STIs because they are linked to sex, and you may worry that people will be judgmental about it. This stigma can make you feel guilty or embarrassed, both for having sex and for contracting an STI. But your sexual health, and that of your partner or partners, should be your top concern. Contracting gonorrhea—or any other STI—does not make you a bad person. Unfortunately, this shame and fear of judgment can keep teens from taking the steps to prevent and treat their STIs.

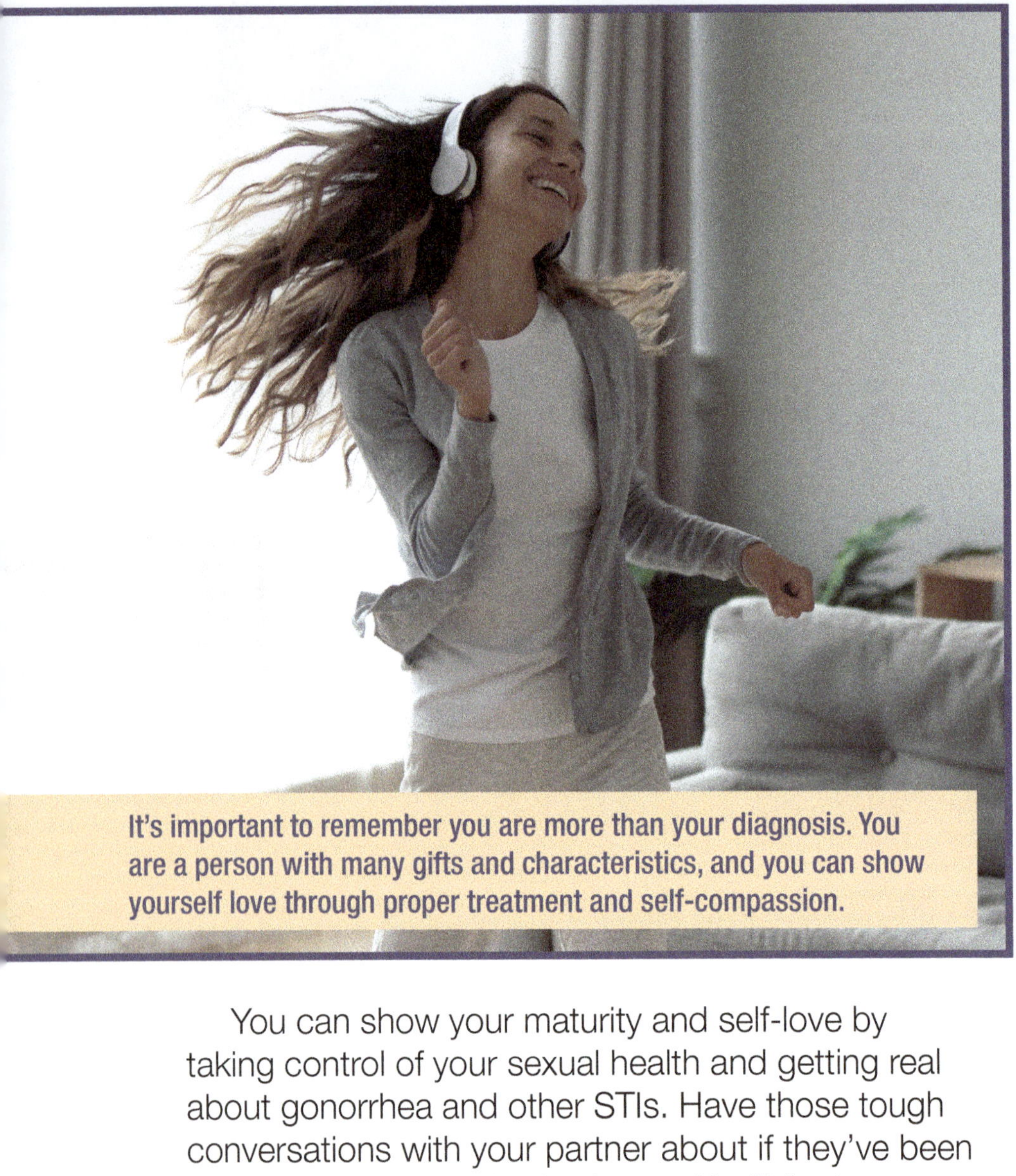

It's important to remember you are more than your diagnosis. You are a person with many gifts and characteristics, and you can show yourself love through proper treatment and self-compassion.

You can show your maturity and self-love by taking control of your sexual health and getting real about gonorrhea and other STIs. Have those tough conversations with your partner about if they've been tested and who they've had sex with. Talk about precautions and educate yourself on how to keep yourself safe and well. And if you contract gonorrhea, you can do what you need to do to get better.

THE CARE YOU NEED

Getting the correct medical care should be your number one priority. Making the doctor's appointment, going to a health clinic, or getting a positive test can also make you feel stressed or depressed. If so, you need to take one more step—find someone to talk to. A parent, teacher, partner, or good friend can help you through your STI diagnosis and treatment. People who are open, loving, and supportive are often the best people to talk with because they care about you and want to help you. Sometimes, however, that isn't possible or you might need more information or support than they are able to give you. The next step is to get some professional mental health counseling.

A mental health counselor can help you to deal with all kinds of emotional and physical challenges and can also help you come to terms with having an STI. Along with making sure you have the necessary information about your condition and helping you understand your treatment options, a good counselor will also talk to you about overcoming feelings of shame, as well as help you make decisions about safer sexual behavior for the future.

Mental health counselors or school counselors can also help you learn coping tools. These tools—such as meditation, breathing exercises, or journaling—can help you deal with hard feelings around stressful situations. You can also learn tools for better communication with those around you, including sexual partners. Getting yourself the care you need is the most important thing you can do in a stressful situation.

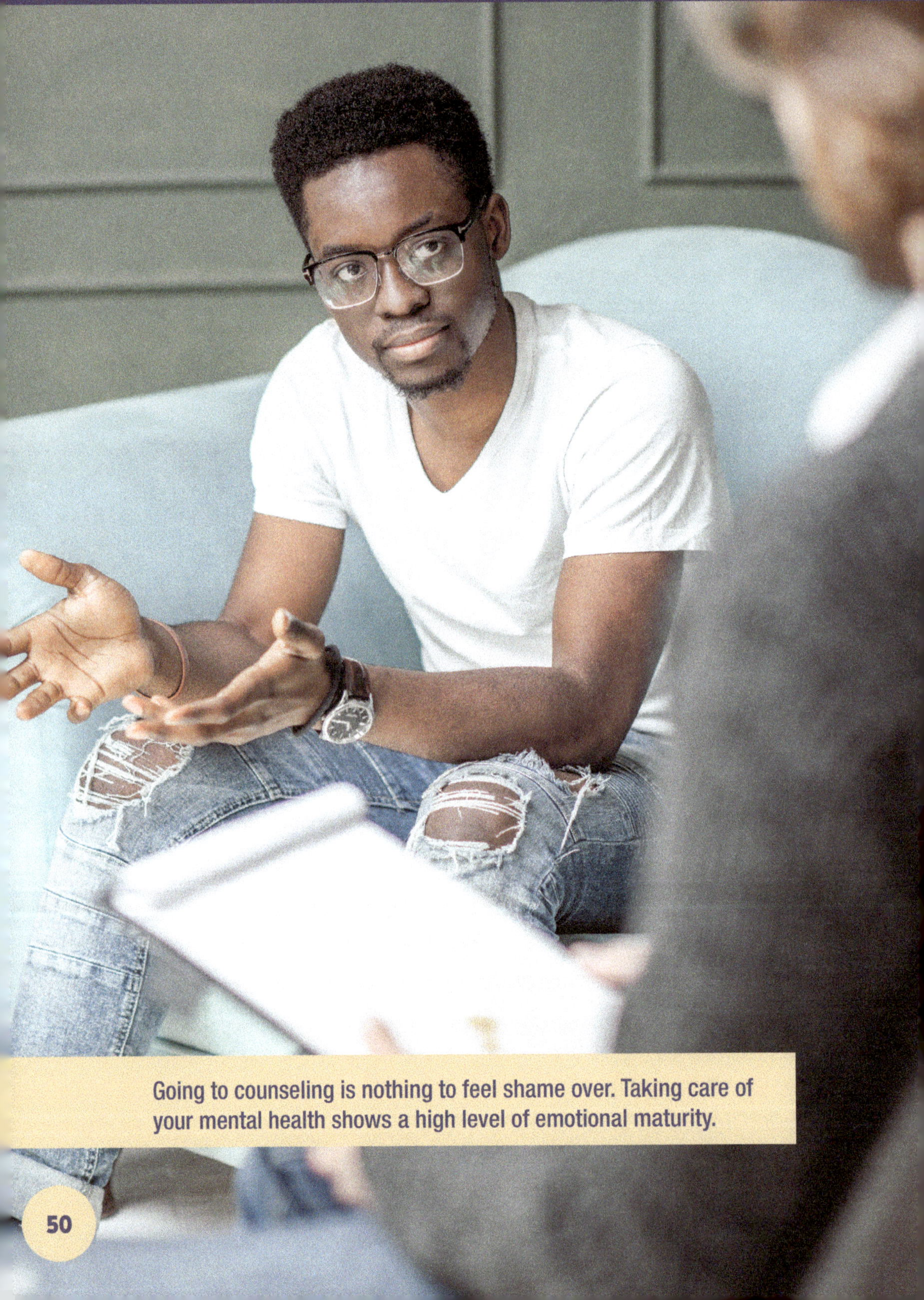

Going to counseling is nothing to feel shame over. Taking care of your mental health shows a high level of emotional maturity.

SHOW YOUR SUPPORT

Maybe you don't have gonorrhea, but someone you know has it. You can be a great support for that person just by showing that you care. Being treated for an STI can be an isolating experience, and people may feel they can't be open about their struggles. You can show your friend or loved one that you are there for them, and that they can talk to you if they want to.

Supporting friends who have an STI is much like supporting them through other life challenges, from other illnesses or injuries to dealing with breakups. You can make sure your loved one realizes how important it is to get proper medical care and treatment. You can educate them on what gonorrhea is, how it's contracted, and how it can affect them if they don't get treatment. If they feel angry, depressed, frustrated, or embarrassed, you can be a shoulder to cry on or a sounding board for their emotions. If they are afraid to go to the doctor or clinic alone, you can offer to go with them for support.

Being a friend means being there for all the laughter and fun times—and all the rough spots as well. Your friendship and support during the testing and treatment of an STI can mean everything to someone. Whether you are the one dealing with gonorrhea or you are the friend who is stepping up to help, it helps to approach the situation with compassion, acceptance, and education.

SUPPORT SYSTEMS

Who supports you when you're going through a difficult time? You might not think about who will be there for you, and who you can depend on, until you're already going through something. But these support systems are important when you're trying to deal with a diagnosis. It's important to set up a system of people you can talk with honestly and without fear of judgment. This can make it easier to accept what's happened, make wise decisions, and follow through with recommended treatment.

You might find it easier to talk to certain people in your family about sex than others, such as siblings, parents, or other family members. You might also be able to talk to friends about it. If you need someone else to talk to, however, there are teen support groups and organizations that can help. Going to a local group where everyone understands what you're going through can be empowering and comforting. You can search online for a local group or check in with your doctor for contact information. Whether you find support through people you know, or people who are just going through the same thing, you can get the comfort and acceptance you deserve.

KNOWLEDGE IS POWER

Learning about STIs gives you power over them—power to prevent the infection, to recognize the symptoms, and to find testing and treatment options. Reading this book is a great start to your STI education. However, you might also want to check out information from reputable online resources too.

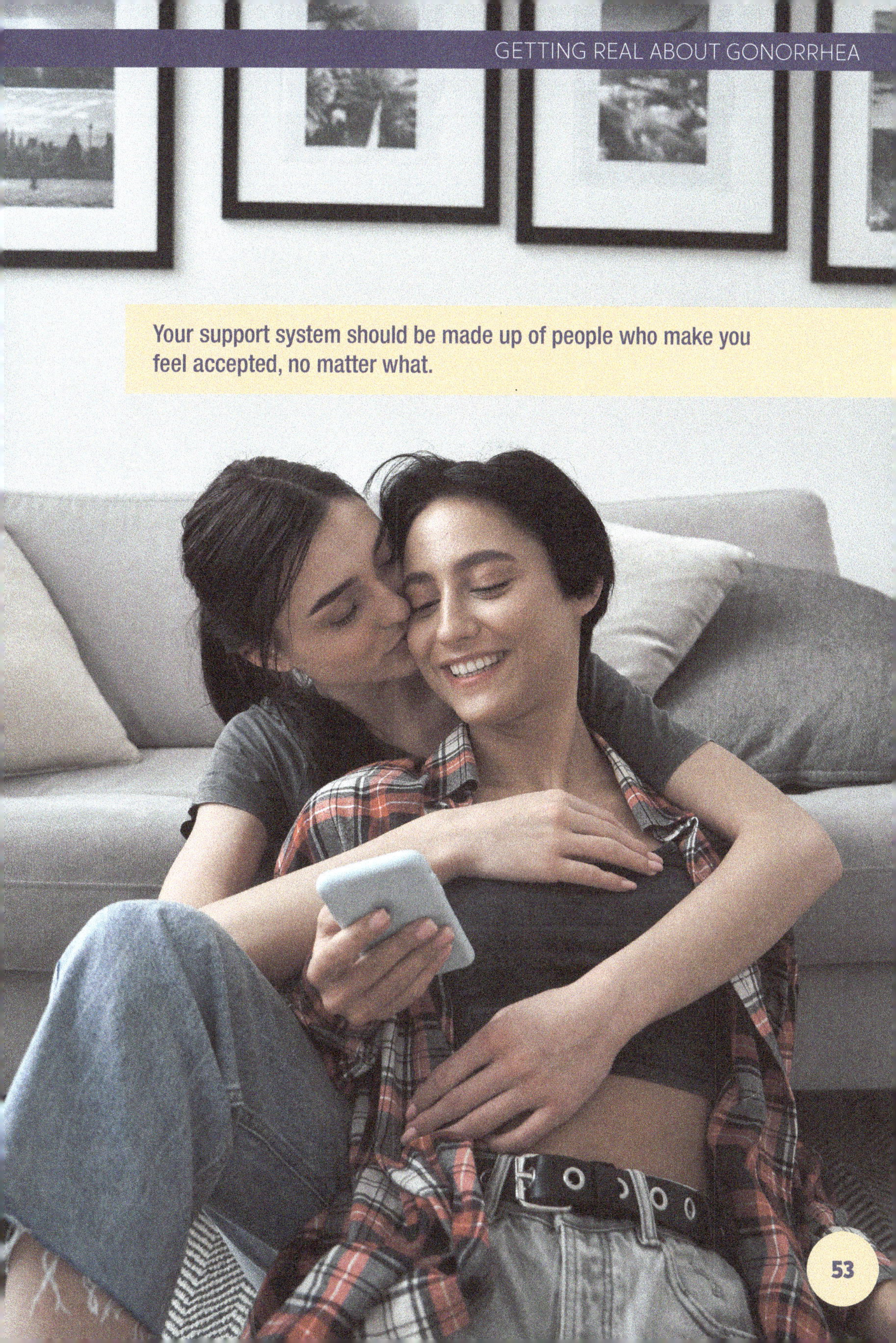

Your support system should be made up of people who make you feel accepted, no matter what.

You might want to join groups online specifically for people with gonorrhea. Remember never to disclose any personal information online and to report anything that makes you uncomfortable.

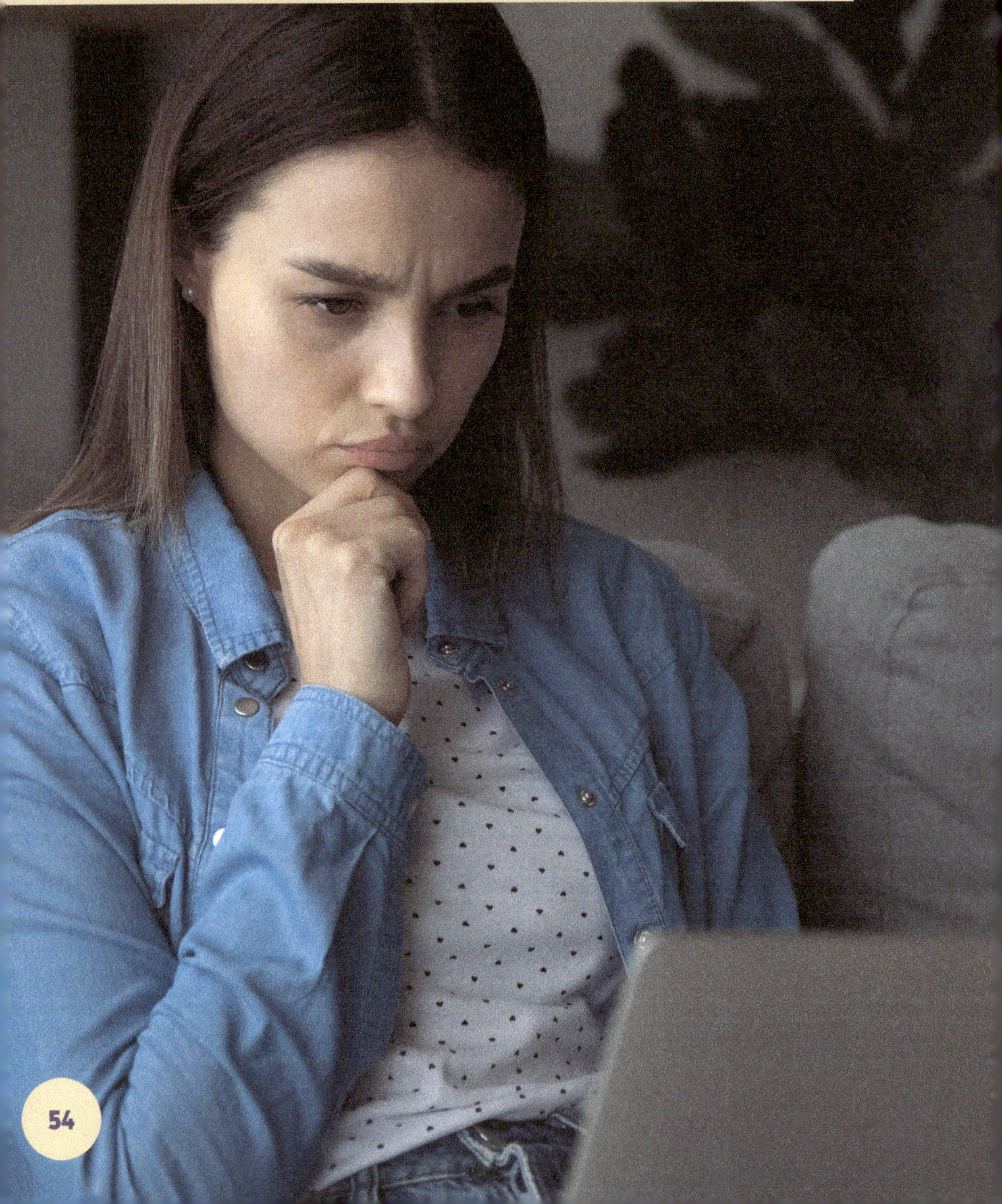

It's important to know which websites have well-researched and correct information, and which websites have misinformation. Reputable websites often end in .org, .edu, or .gov. You may notice that an article in a news source was written by a doctor, and that can mean it's got accurate information too. You should never try to diagnose yourself based on information from websites alone. Always check with a medical professional about your diagnosis and treatment. Chat threads about a certain alternative remedy or treatment may lead you to try unhelpful, and sometimes harmful, things.

You can fight gonorrhea with the most powerful tool there is—knowledge. It is a curable STI, and it is also a preventable one. Give yourself the best shot to beat gonorrhea with accurate information, a great support system, and respect for your sexual health.

GLOSSARY

abstinence The practice of abstaining from something, or not doing something that is wanted or enjoyable.

brothel A building in which prostitutes, or people paid for sex, are available.

contraception Methods of birth control to prevent pregnancy.

dental dam A square sheet of rubber that can be used in dentistry and oral sex.

ejaculate The ejection of semen from a male body at the moment of sexual climax.

epididymis The coiled tubes in the back of the testicles.

genitalia External reproductive organs.

immune Having a high degree of resistance to a disease.

infertility Incapable of or unsuccessful in achieving pregnancy.

inflammation A response in the body to injury or illness that's marked by redness, heat, and pain.

inhibition The mental process of putting restraint upon behavior or desire.

lubricant A substance used for minimizing friction during sexual intercourse.

meningitis Inflammation of the brain lining caused by a viral or bacterial infection.

misinformation Incorrect or misleading information.

monogamy The practice of being with only one sexual partner at a time.

mucous membrane A tissue that secretes mucus and lines body cavities including the stomach and respiratory passages.

pandemic An outbreak of disease that occurs over a wide geographic area and affects a great proportion of the population.

pelvic adhesions Bands of scar tissue that may cause internal organs to stick to one another, such as the ovaries or uterus.

precaution A measure taken beforehand to prevent harm.

semen A fluid of the male reproductive tract that contains spermatozoa, which is capable of fertilizing the egg of a female.

serum A fluid obtained from the blood of an individual who has recovered from an infectious disease and may contain antibodies against the infectious agent of the disease.

spermicide A substance that kills sperm and can be used as a contraceptive or with another contraceptive.

susceptible Vulnerable to contracting a disease.

symptom Something that indicates the existence of a certain disease or condition.

topical Applied to the skin.

urethra The duct by which urine is carried out of the body from the bladder; in males, it also conveys semen.

venereologist A person who specializes in studying sexually transmitted diseases.

FOR MORE INFORMATION

Advocates for Youth
1325 G Street NW, Suite 980
Washington, DC 20005
Website: www.advocatesforyouth.org
Instagram: @advocatesforyouth
Twitter: @AdvocatesTweets
Advocates for Youth focuses on building youth power through sexual health and education.

American Sexual Health Association (ASHA)
P.O. Box 13827
Research Triangle Park, NC 27709
Website: www.ashasexualhealth.org
Instagram: @ashasexualhealth
Twitter: @InfoASHA
ASHA has worked for over 100 years to improve the sexual health of individuals, families, and communities through providing STD education, support, and advocacy.

Healthy Teen Network
1501 Saint Paul Street, Suite 114
Baltimore, MD 21202
Website: www.healthyteennetwork.org
Instagram: @healthyteennetwork
Twitter: @healthyteen
This organization works to advance social change, connect teens, and empower teens to protect their health and be more aware of sexual health issues.

National Coalition for Sexual Health
Website: nationalcoalitionforsexualhealth.org/contact
Instagram: @nationalcoalitionsexualhealth
Twitter: @NCSH_
This coalition works together to improve the sexual health of Americans, make sexual health a part of normal conversation, and spread accurate sexual health information.

Planned Parenthood
Phone: 1-800-230-PLAN
Website: www.plannedparenthood.org
Instagram: @plannedparenthood
Twitter: @PPFA
Planned Parenthood is a nonprofit organization that provides sexual and reproductive healthcare, sexual education, and accurate information on sexual health to people around the world.

FOR FURTHER READING

DeCarlo, Carolyn. *Everything You Need to Know About the Risks of Unprotected Sex.* New York, NY: Rosen Publishing, 2019.

Gonzales, Katheryn, and and Karen Rayne PhD *Trans+: Love, Sex, Romance, and Being You*. Washington, DC: Magination Press, 2019.

Harris, Robie H. *It's Perfectly Normal: Changing Bodies, Growing Up, Sex, Gender, and Sexual Health.* Somerville, MA: Candlewick Press, 2021.

Hope, Michelle, and Amy Lang. *The Girls' Guide to Sex Education: Over 100 Honest Answers to Urgent Questions about Puberty, Relationships, and Growing Up*. Emeryville, CA: Rockridge Press, 2018.

Lang, Jennifer. *Consent: The New Rules of Sex Education: Every Teen's Guide to Healthy Sexual Relationships*. San Antonio, TX: Althea Press, 2018.

Langford, Jo. *The Pride Guide: A Guide to Sexual and Social Health for LGBTQ Youth.* Lanham, MD: Rowman & Littlefield, 2018.

Moem, Erika, and Matthew Nolan. *Let's Talk About It: The Teen's Guide to Sex, Relationships, and Being a Human*. New York, NY: Random House Graphic, 2021.

Parrish, Jacqueline. *Coping with Sexually Transmitted Diseases.* New York, NY: Rosen Young Adult, 2019.

Planned Parenthood. *In Case You're Curious: Questions About Sex from Young People with Answers from the Experts.* Berkeley, CA: Viva Editions, 2019.

Wolny, Philip. *I Have an STD. Now What?* New York, NY: Rosen Publishing, 2015.

INDEX